Praise for
The Ultimate College Student Health Handbook

"Over the years, I have learned that the typical college student with a health concern will generally consult their roommate or Dr. Google in lieu of seeking help from an actual physician. Not only does Dr. Grimes give expert advice of what to do about common college ailments, but even more important, she is clear about when getting medical attention is not optional. *The Ultimate College Student Health Handbook* is the next best thing to having your own family doctor as your college student's roommate. Other than paying tuition, this is the most valuable gift you can give a student."
—**Lauren Streicher, MD, Clinical Professor of Ob-Gyn,**
Northwestern University, Chicago, IL

"As a pediatrician and child health expert, parents look to me for trusted advice. I wholeheartedly recommend *The Ultimate College Student Health Handbook*, an accurate, practical guide that will help your kids deal with unexpected illnesses, injuries, and anxieties (and will give you answers for their late-night texts). Definitely my new go-to high school graduation gift!"
—**Tanya Remer Altmann, MD, bestselling author and parenting expert**

"A healthy body and a healthy mind! Dr. Jill Grimes skillfully addresses the vast array of college woes, from sore throat to STIs, recognizes the ills anxiety can cause, and has the answers to young adults' health questions that will carry them through a lifetime. Buy this for your college student . . . and maybe even yourself!"
—**Sanjiv Chopra, MD, MACP, bestselling author**
and professor of Medicine at Harvard Medical School

"This is an essential guide to health and wellness when you head off to college . . . and your mom can't be there to hold your hand and take care of you."
—**Ari Brown, MD, FAAP, bestselling author of Baby 411 series**

"A graduation gift that will give for a lifetime! *The Ultimate College Student Health Handbook* is the most important book your college-bound child needs to take to school. . . . A gift as much for the parent as the college-bound student, this book is truly First Aid for Adulthood. With her years of experience in college health, Dr. Jill Grimes summarizes the common conditions we worry about, explains how to help treat the symptoms, and advises as to when to visit the health center. Dr. Grimes debunks myths and touches on the key points parents want their adult children to know (but often cannot find the words to say) in clear and insightful terms."

—Frank J. Domino, MD, professor at the University of Massachusetts Medical School, Dept. of Family Medicine and Community Health, editor-in-chief of *5-Minute Clinical Consult*

"Every college freshman needs a copy of *The Ultimate College Student Health Handbook*! This book addresses the most common medical issues encountered in the college years and teaches your student how to handle them like a champ . . . without having to call Mom or Dad for advice. Written by a University Health Center family doctor with years of experience who's seen it all, this book will also help parents feel confident that their college student's health is in good hands."

—Gretchen LaSalle, MD, MultiCare Rockwood Clinic Family Medicine, author of *Let's Talk Vaccines: A Clinician's Guide to Addressing Vaccine Hesitancy and Saving Lives*

"Dr. Grimes has done it again! She's been a favorite speaker for both teens and parents for years, and now we are thrilled to have her college survival skills neatly packaged in a book to send off with our kids as they fly the nest! The Ultimate College Student Health Handbook is the perfect gift for every high school graduate. The format makes health issues easy to look up and each section gives great 'tips' for prevention and maintaining a healthy lifestyle. I especially appreciate the inclusion of mental health issues such as depression and panic disorder!"

—Kimberly Snyder, MD, FACEP, Emergency Medicine Physician, Past President Capital of Texas Chapter of National Charity League

"Parents should buy two copies of this book—one for themselves and one for their college-bound teenager!"

—**Julie K. Silver, MD, associate professor, Harvard Medical School**

"Within the pages of this book—the one you're contemplating reading this very moment—lies no ordinary how-to. First, because Dr. Jill Grimes successfully tackles most—and I mean that!—common teenage ailments. Second, because she takes a refreshingly entertaining approach in doing it. The result? A book I'd recommend to ANY parent who wants a quick reference on hand for those what-could-the-doctor-say moments."

—**Dana Corriel, MD, SoMeDocs Founder & CEO,**
Top 10 Internists to Follow on Twitter, Medical Economics,
Top 20 Physician Influencers on Social Media, Medscape

"Wow! As a registered dietitian and past president of Austin Aggie Moms, I wish I would have had such a phenomenal resource to hand to my children when they set out for college. From acne to UTIs, Dr. Grimes's book covers all the basics of health care for any college student. I heartily recommend it to moms, students, and former students!"

—**Daniela R. Knight, MS, RD, LD, board member of the**
Federation of Texas A&M University Mothers' Clubs

"I SO wish we had this book to give our son when we sent him off to college a few months ago (but he'll have one now!). Once again, Dr. Grimes has written an extremely practical guide for parents and young adults alike, brilliantly organized and easy to reference the most frequent health concerns for college students. She candidly approaches each subject with clarity and compassion, much the same way she discusses these types of topics in person. Dr. Grimes is a favorite local speaker with mothers and daughters in NCL and mothers and sons in the Young Men's Service League (YMSL), and we are all thrilled she has now packaged up her wisdom to share with everyone. If you're the parent of a college-bound student, buy several for graduation gifts. If you're a college student, get this book to make the 'best years of your life' even better!"

—**Dianne Field, president, Capitol of Texas**
Chapter of National Charity League

THE ULTIMATE
College
Student
Health
HANDBOOK

Your Guide for Everything from
HANGOVERS to HOMESICKNESS

THIRD EDITION

Jill Grimes, MD, FAAFP

Illustrations by **Nicole Grimes**

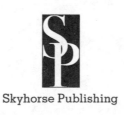

Skyhorse Publishing

To our favorite college students,
Brittany & Nicole,
And to "Ye Old Prof," their beloved Grandpap,
who taught us from an early age,
"If you didn't fall, you weren't trying!"

Text copyright © 2020, 2022, 2024 by Jill Grimes
Illustrations copyright © 2020, 2022, 2024 by Nicole Grimes

Skyhorse Publishing books may be purchased in bulk at special discounts for sales promotion, corporate gifts, fund-raising, or educational purposes. Special editions can also be created to specifications. For details, contact the Special Sales Department, Skyhorse Publishing, 307 West 36th Street, 11th Floor, New York, NY 10018 or info@skyhorsepublishing.com.

Skyhorse® and Skyhorse Publishing® are registered trademarks of Skyhorse Publishing, Inc.®, a Delaware corporation.

Visit our website at www.skyhorsepublishing.com.

10 9 8 7 6 5 4 3

Library of Congress Cataloging-in-Publication Data is available on file.

Cover design by Daniel Brount
Cover illustration credit: Nicole Grimes
Editor: Nicole Frail

Print ISBN: 978-1-5107-7889-4
Ebook ISBN: 978-1-5107-5105-7

Printed in the United States of America

Note to the Reader

This book is not meant to be a substitute for medical care, and treatment should not be based solely on these recommendations because each person has a unique medical history, including medication allergies, prior surgeries, and chronic illnesses such as diabetes or asthma, etc. This book was written to help college students understand more about different physical and emotional symptoms (and what ailments those symptoms might suggest), as well as to learn what to expect during an evaluation from a medical professional. The information provided here does not constitute a doctor-patient relationship between the author and the reader. Views and content are Dr. Grimes's and do not necessarily represent those of her employers, past or present.

This book presents many "what-if" scenarios that share typical stories of young people with these issues that occur on every college campus, none of which portray any single individual; any resemblance to a specific person whom Dr. Grimes has treated is coincidental.

Medications have been identified by their generic name followed by at least one brand name in parentheses, but this is intended to be neither a comprehensive list of all possible brands nor all prescription or over-the-counter options. The author has made reasonable efforts to apply current evidence-based medical recommendations for all treatments described in this book, but given ongoing research and constantly evolving information regarding drug therapy, the reader is encouraged to talk with their doctor and pharmacist regarding specific doses, warnings, and precautions.

Contents

Preface

Congratulations! If you've picked up this book, odds are great that either you or someone important in your life has been **accepted to college** and is heading off for the next chapter in their life. How exciting . . . and, at the same time, how scary, unknown, and possibly nerve-racking!

If you are a PARENT (especially if this is kid #1 launching), you may find yourself frantically cramming in every bit of last-minute advice you might possibly have forgotten to dispense during the last eighteen years. *Can you tell I've been there, done that?* I successfully resisted the temptation to completely bubble-wrap our girls as they each flew in different directions over a thousand miles away from the nest. However, as a **doctor mom**, I did at least send them off with a fully stocked first aid kit and personalized instruction booklet that I had been perfecting over the past decade (it was my high school graduation gift of choice). Those instructions began with basic advice for dealing with ailments like food poisoning, heartburn, homesickness, hangovers, and even choice of pain medicine (when to take Tylenol versus Advil). Each year, I added more topics until that booklet evolved into the book you now hold.

If you are a STUDENT, again—**congrats!** You are totally ready and prepared **enough** for college, I promise. We all know how hard it is to get into universities these days, so if you are accepted, you are **smart** and **ready**. Does that mean you won't have bad days? Of course not! **When (not if) you get sick or anxious, it's going to be a bad day** . . . or maybe a bad week. I hope this book can be a quick reference and starting point for you on those tough days, so you have a better idea what to expect about your problem. My goal is for you to understand if and when you really need to see a doctor (on or off campus) to be fully evaluated and treated.

How do I know what college students REALLY want (or need) to know? I keep my finger on the pulse of young adults, both in person and across social media platforms, especially as the TikTok CollegeDoc. Meanwhile, our kids and their continually expanding network of friends happily still text me questions without fear of judgment or violation of their privacy. After twenty years of taking care of families in private practice, I followed my heart and passion and switched practice settings to exclusively treat college students as patients for the next seven years at the University of Texas. Truth be told, I'm a proud Texas Aggie (Class of '87, whoop!) which happens to be the Longhorns' traditional rival. During my years at UT, I loved sharing laughs and good-natured teasing when students noticed my Aggie ring and shared their favorite Aggie jokes. At the end of the day, I know what college students want and need to know, because they literally tell me . . . and I hear the same concerns, fears, and questions over and over again.

What are students worried about? Everything! Newfound anxiety over tests, public speaking, or common bathrooms; heartburn or emotional heartache; sprained ankles or painful knees; road rash or concussions; first-time stomach flu away from home; incapacitating migraines; or even first-semester FOMO (Fear of Missing Out)-induced homesickness. **My goal is to offer a quick reference guide beyond "Dr. Google" for both the students** themselves and their **concerned parents,** who might be unsure how to answer that late-night text.

This book is not intended to be a *"sit down and read it cover-to-cover"* book, but instead a handy reference, organized literally head to toe by the primary body part affected. As such, there is some overlap and repetition between topics, because I'm assuming you are reading them on different days, months, or years. For example, Cognitive Behavioral Therapy (CBT) is briefly explained in multiple topics because CBT happens to be an excellent, effective, and specific type of talk-therapy/counseling that is the treatment of choice for multiple concerns from fear of public restrooms or test anxiety to insomnia and even nail-biting.

I've made every effort to apply Evidence-Based Medicine (EBM) in this book. This means that the diagnostic and treatment recommendations are based upon high-quality, non-biased research studies that examine clinical outcomes and consider the patient's values and preferences. For example, most backaches and ankle sprains do *not* require X-rays, and the majority of sinus infections, bronchitis, and coughs will *not* improve with antibiotics! **Parents, *please stop telling your student to "go in and get an X-ray" or "go get antibiotics."*** I swear (we literally take the Hippocratic Oath, remember?) that we want to heal every patient as much as they and you want them to feel better. Writing an antibiotic prescription for bronchitis (which is usually viral) may make us all feel like we are "doing something," but the evidence shows doing so offers the patient more risk of harm than true help (because of medication side effects or, at a minimum, wallet drain). My hope is that by including and explaining EBM recommendations in different topics, students (and their parents) will have more accurate diagnostic and treatment **expectations**. This knowledge will enhance communication and build confidence as your student learns to navigate the health care system on their own.

Which topics are included? Medicine is not so simple that I can cover every possible college-aged health issue, so I primarily chose the most common complaints. A few topics are included, however, because students don't know what they don't know . . . like that chest pain without an injury could be a partially collapsed lung or a blood clot. Most topics begin with the universal stories that students share about "what probably happened," but a few subjects jump directly to my standard exam-room conversational Q&A: Stimulants 101 (ADHD Meds, Risks, and Mistakes); Smoking, Vaping, and What You Might Not Know About Pot; Freshman Fifteen, and Thinking of Inking? Tattoos (Before and After).

What is not included? While this book addresses Sexually Transmitted Infections (STIs), they are not the main focus, and writing on each individually creates another book. Which I've already written. Twice. Therefore, after a decade of talking with young people and writing on this ever-important but awkward topic, I chose to combine all the Sexually Transmitted

Infections (Yes, It Happens to People like You) into a few scenarios of "what probably happened" along with the critical take-home messages, in my own version of STI "SparkNotes®." And while pregnancy prevention is addressed, ectopic (tubal) and other unexpected outcomes are not. Likewise, gender identity and sexual preference issues are not specifically discussed, because while these complex topics are certainly part of college health, there is not space in this book to adequately address these topics. I therefore respectfully refer you to the steadily growing collection of excellent books and resources devoted solely to these critical and challenging subjects. Please know I have consciously alternated or used gender-neutral pronouns (he/she/they), and I sought, received, and incorporated feedback from a cross-section of under-represented groups in a sincere attempt for inclusivity.

What's new this edition? "Know Before You Go: 12 Tips for Doctor Visits (On Your Own)" will help students plow through the intimidating insurance and medical paperwork, plus learn strategies for more effective and efficient communication with their clinicians. (Take note, parents!) We also added "Seizures," which are far more common than you might expect, plus the potentially lifesaving "One Pill Can Kill: How to Recognize and Treat Opioid (Fentanyl) Overdose," which also shares why and how smart, "good" kids end up needing this knowledge.

Many college students (up to a third of college undergrads) *choose not to drink alcohol, smoke, vape, try other people's prescription stimulants or even street drugs, get tattoos, and/or have sex,* while many others are comfort-able with any or all these choices. Rest assured, this book is not a how-to manual designed to strongly encourage risky decisions. There is also no intention to condescendingly shame anyone for their choices. **College students are independent young adults learning to balance decisions and consequences, and the reality is that these issues exist on every college campus.** My sincere hope is that these topics offer a nonjudgmental*, medically relevant, and informative conversation starter.

---

* Full disclosure, I am extremely antismoking, antivaping, and obviously anti-prescription or street drug abuse. My patients who choose these high-risk behaviors know I will kindly but mercilessly reeducate them each and every visit.

Finally, while I hate that our legal climate makes me use disclaimers saying this is not official medical advice, and that you (or your son/daughter) are not my patient, that's the world we live in. Every person brings their own medical history, which can potentially affect any diagnosis or treatment, and I obviously don't have the benefit of examining you. This is the very ART of medicine, after all! However, this book does offer information that should help you (the student) feel more confident as you learn to independently navigate your college health-care system and interact with new physicians and other providers.

Parents, what can I say? This is definitely not bubble wrap, but I hope sending this book (along with the suggested DIY first aid kit) off to college with your student gives you some sense of reassurance that your awesome daughter or son has a trustworthy starting point when they are injured, ill, or anxious. We see your kids at their most exhausted, most frustrated, sickest worst, yet I'm here to tell you that they are consistently respectful, polite, and far more "adult" than you would imagine, even when they are scared or hurting. So, congrats to you, too, because you've done a great job raising them, and they are ready for this next step! And on those days when they are injured, sick, or anxious, we (in college health across the country) are here—ready, willing, and able to help.

Students, Welcome to College! The next several years typically offer the most freedom coupled with the least responsibility that you will enjoy as an adult, which is a big reason people say college will be "the best years of your life." Challenge yourself to use that precious time to absorb the full college experience in and out of the classroom, taking advantage of campus theater, sports, clubs, politics, music, social justice, volunteering, or whatever inspires you, and these years will be indeed be great. *I wish you a fabulous, safe, and healthy collegiate journey!*

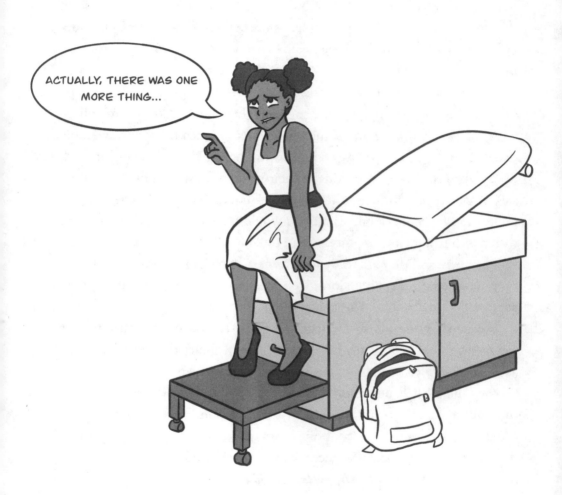

Know Before You Go: 12 Tips for Doctor Visits (On Your Own)

Most college students have not yet had to deal with the logistics of health care—all the health insurance forms, medical history paperwork, and, yes, the complicated payments. Although an adult you trust may only be a quick text away, here are a dozen things you should know before you head to your first solo doctor appointment:

1. **TAKE A PICTURE OF YOUR HEALTH INSURANCE CARD NOW** (both front and back) and "favorite" it on your phone. Also, create an easily accessible document (like Google Doc) that includes this insurance card photo along with all the other health information suggested below. The very first thing any medical receptionist or pharmacy will ask for is your health insurance card. If you don't have the actual card with you, most places will let you email them that picture of your card and they can print it out.

2. **HEALTH INSURANCE CARD INFORMATION CAN BE MORE CONFUSING THAN YOU WOULD EXPECT.** Here is what to look for on the card when you are filling out medical forms:

Front:

○ **Member/Subscriber Name** (this is the person that enrolled in the plan and pays the monthly premiums, typically your parent/guardian, not you)

○ **Dependents** (this includes you if you're on someone else's insurance plan)

○ **ID number** (a.k.a. "Member ID," which is your family's specific identification number)

○ **Group Number** (this number is unique to the company offering the health insurance, i.e., the insured's employer)

○ **Copay amounts** tell you how much you pay immediately up front, for example:

- Office visit with your primary care provider: $10*
- Office visit with a specialist: $30*
- Emergency room visit: $100*
- Prescription medications: $10 generic/$30 for brand name/$50 "other"**

  amounts listed above obviously vary with different insurance policies

  ** "Other" means specific, more expensive medications that your insurance covers partially, but you pay a greater amount. *Note that not every medication is covered, so at times you may have to pay full price despite having insurance.*

If you are shocked at the cost of your prescription, you may decline the medication and have the pharmacist (or yourself) check back with your doctor about possibly prescribing an alternative, less expensive drug. Medication prices may vary significantly by pharmacy, so also consider checking the price at a few different pharmacy chains or locations. Insurance companies, pharmacy benefit managers, and pharmaceutical companies negotiate contracts that ultimately set medication costs for the consumer, with each insurance company creating a "formulary"—a list of preferred medications. With the multitude of insurance offerings and frequent formulary changes (as contracts expire and are renegotiated), your physician may have no idea what your specific cost will be for a given prescription. Occasionally, it even costs less to buy a prescription medication without using your insurance because the drug (typically a generic) price is less than your copay. **Drug prices are confusing and frustrating for all of us!** The bottom line is that the ONLY way we know that a medication was too expensive for you (or not covered by your insurance) is for you to reach back and tell us. *Please do not wait until your follow-up visit to tell us you never purchased the medication we prescribed, or that you did purchase it, but it was insanely expensive!*

Back: your insurance company's contact information
○ Phone numbers for customer service reps (for you and for your medical providers)
○ Mailing address—for billing purposes

3. **GUARANTOR:** When you are filling out the business paperwork, they will ask for a "GUARANTOR." his is the person ultimately RESPONSIBLE FOR PAYING THE BILL. *For college students who are still on their parent/guardian's health insurance, the guarantor is typically the person listed as the member on your health insurance card.* NOTE: Forms often require the guarantor's social security number (so find that out now and store it in a safe, convenient place on your phone, like in your password keeper or on a Google doc if your parent/guardian is comfortable with that.)

4. **PRIVACY:** Once you are eighteen, medical providers cannot and will not discuss your care with anyone else unless you specifically ask them to do so AND sign a consent/release form. Be aware, however, that insurance statements called "Explanation of Benefits" (EOBs) will be sent to the "primary enrollee" of the

insurance plan, which for students on their parent/guardian's health insurance plan, will be that person. While the EOB does not contain any diagnoses, it does spell out what procedures and tests were run. *Translation: if you are not comfortable talking with anyone in your family about issues like testing for pregnancy or sexually transmittable diseases, think about this before you choose to pay with your family's insurance.*

5. **IMMUNIZATION RECORD:** Take a photo or manually add your immunization record to your health document, and highlight your last tetanus shot, because that is a very common vaccination asked about in urgent care (typically for "dirty" injuries like stepping on a nail). When you get your annual flu shot (much encouraged!), be sure to add that to your phone calendar and/or your document for easy reference. Ditto for all other immunizations.

6. **MEDICATION LIST**: Add a complete list of your medications to your health document, including either the generic or brand name, plus the dose. Many people find it helpful to include a description, ex: Fluoxetine 20 mg, one pill each morning (antidepressant, generic for Prozac). Be sure to include prescription medications that you use "as needed" such as asthma inhalers or migraine medicines. If you take any over-the-counter medications regularly, add those to the list (like nasal steroids sprays for allergies, melatonin, vitamins, etc.).

7. **ALLERGIES to MEDICATIONS:** List which medications (especially antibiotics) and what kind of reaction you had—was it a total body rash or an "anaphylactic" emergency?

8. **FAMILY HISTORY:** Many diseases with a familial predisposition start showing up during college years. Note what runs in your family, *especially diseases present in multiple and/or immediate family members.* Some we see more commonly include kidney stones, gallstones, depression, diabetes, migraines, colitis, autoimmune diseases, anemia, bipolar disorder, and certain cancers.

9. **SURGERIES:** Yes, we even want to know if you had ear tubes as a baby! Have you had your tonsils removed? Appendix? Wisdom teeth? Knee or shoulder surgeries? Were you born with a serious heart abnormality that was surgically corrected? Again, add all these to your accessible health document.

10. **BE HONEST**. We are not asking about how much alcohol you drink, or whether you smoke/vape/use THC products or other illegal substances to be nosy or get you in trouble. We ask because these substances can negatively impact your health (for example, they may cause insomnia or stomach pain) and/or they may interact with a medication we want to prescribe for you. Ditto for any detailed questions about your sexual history—this is typically to assess your risk for different sexually transmittable infections.

11. **DOCTORS OFTEN REPEAT QUESTIONS** you may have already answered multiple times during your pre-appointment questionnaire or with the medical assistant who brought you in to the exam room and took your vital signs. We know this can feel incredibly frustrating and sometimes even offensive (appearing that we do not believe your answer). *Why do we do it?* Sometimes, we ask because it is honestly faster to repeat the question than to look through the records. Most of the time, it is simply part of our thinking process as we clarify certain details. Lastly, the truth is that patients often change their answers about sensitive topics, largely because they did not feel comfortable sharing the full details initially, for a variety of reasons. So yes, sometimes we choose to repeat a question to be sure the first answer was accurate, but not in a judgmental way.

12. **LEAD WITH YOUR MOST PRESSING CONCERN.** When you book your appointment, you are given a set amount of time for your visit based on what you say is your primary issue. Flu symptoms or an injured ankle may be given a ten-minute appointment, for example, while insomnia and depression may be allotted twice that time. Many people wait till the doctor's hand is literally on the doorknob at the end of the visit before

they manage to blurt out why they *really* made the appointment, "Hey, doctor, actually, there was one more thing I wanted to ask!" These "doorknob" questions are typically complex, often a serious concern about a mental or sexual health issue that we really want and need to address, but which may be difficult or impossible given the reality of time limits (and in fairness to the other patients still waiting to be seen). Obviously, if your problem is life-threatening or truly time-sensitive, we will sit back down and address it. *On that note, please be patient when we run behind, because this happens quite frequently.* To maximize the time and attention we can give your concerns, the more direct you can be initially, the better. I give you my word that especially in college health, we hear "embarrassing" concerns all day, every day, and virtually nothing you share will shock your physician. Please do not feel afraid, embarrassed, or ashamed to ask us anything. We are here to help.

Chapter 1
Hangovers

What If: I Have a Hangover?
Medical Name: Headache and Alcohol Toxicity

What most likely happened:
You remember having a couple of beers to settle your nerves when you got to the party last night, and later, everyone was doing shots . . . but the rest is a blur. Now it is 10 a.m., and you've vomited a few times in your dorm room. Your head is threatening to explode, and your gut isn't far behind. Roommates are telling you to drink water and take Advil, but despite being incredibly thirsty, you can't keep anything down.

What's going on?
Obviously, drinking too much alcohol causes hangovers—you know that. Surprisingly, however, scientists are still unclear on the specifics. Here's what we do know:

- **Alcohol is a diuretic (makes you pee).** The body's regulatory antidiuretic hormone (which tells the kidneys **not** to make urine) gets turned off or at least is suppressed by alcohol, which subsequently turns the kidneys "on" to produce more urine. The more urine you make, the more you pee, and then your body reacts to that fluid loss. Dehydration for any reason can cause headaches, muscle aches, and light-headedness—especially when you go from lying down to sitting up, or sitting to standing.

- **Alcohol triggers vasodilation**—swelling of your blood vessels (picture people flushing when they drink)—which then aggravates positional dizziness and causes headaches.
- **Alcohol upsets your stomach in two ways:**
  - Direct irritation of the stomach lining
  - Delayed emptying of the stomach and increased acid production (which causes nausea and vomiting)
- **Alcohol makes your heart race**
  - Dehydration and blood vessel dilation make your heart work harder to circulate less fluid through more space.
- **Alcohol is a sedative**
  - Although alcohol makes you feel sleepy, it messes up your quality of sleep, leaving you feeling extra tired or "brain foggy" the next morning.
- **Alcohol can lower blood sugar levels**
  - Low blood sugar makes you feel shaky, weak, tired, and headachy.
- **Congeners may increase the severity of hangovers**
  - "Congeners" are chemical breakdown products of alcohol metabolism.
  - Dark liquors (like bourbon) contain more "congeners" than light or clear liquors (like vodka).
- **Alcohol triggers an inflammatory response from the immune system** that may be responsible for some of the cloudy thinking, headaches, and muscle aches of a hangover.

Treatment:

Despite miracle products claiming to prevent or cure hangovers, the only answers are hydration, pain relief, and time.

- Nausea can often be helped with OTC antacids (like TUMS or Maalox), but sometimes prescription antinausea medications

such as ondansetron (Zofran) or promethazine (Phenergan) are needed.
- If the nausea is controlled, steadily sip on room-temperature water or a sports drink from a cup (don't use straws).
- When you can tolerate food, try some simple or complex carbohydrates like crackers, a granola bar, or toast before you try to take any pain relievers.
- A broth-based (not creamy) soup can help you both rehydrate and retain fluid because of high salt content.
- Over-the-counter pain relievers can help your head- and muscle aches, but know that ibuprofen and aspirin are irritating to the stomach (so not a great choice if you are nauseated) and acetaminophen (Tylenol) can irritate the liver and must be used with extreme caution if you regularly drink heavily.
- If you still can't rehydrate despite prescription antinausea medicines, *you may need IV fluids to rehydrate adequately.*

Head to your doctor if you are:
- Trying to sip on water or a sports drink, but you keep vomiting for over an hour.
- Incapacitated by the severity of your headache.

Worst-case scenario:
Do not confuse an awake, alert, sober, but nauseated and hungover person with someone who is acutely intoxicated and vomiting from alcohol poisoning. *Hangovers occur when blood alcohol levels fade to zero—many hours after drinking stops.* Alcohol poisoning causes vomiting while blood alcohol levels are still high, and that person may have a decreased gag reflex (which increases the chance of choking while vomiting) as well as decreased or irregular breathing, confusion, or loss of consciousness. *This person needs immediate medical attention.* (See Chapter 9: Passed Out: Alcohol Poisoning, page 53.)

Prevention:

Obviously, hangovers only happen if you drink alcohol, so **not** drinking is 100 percent guaranteed to prevent this problem. However, a few things will decrease your risk of a hangover IF you decide to drink:

- **Never drink on an empty stomach**, because an empty stomach absorbs alcohol more quickly.
- **Don't drink while ADHD medications are in your system**, because you won't feel the normal signs of alcohol building up in your system.
  - See Chapter 8: Stimulants 101 (ADHD Meds, Risks, and Mistakes) (page 48).
- **Drink beer, wine, or wine coolers** (*rather than doing shots*).
  - Yes, you **can** get alcohol toxicity and/or severe hangovers from beer or wine, *but you have to really work at it!* And **no,** I'm not encouraging that but pointing out that when we see purely beer-induced alcohol toxicity, virtually every time that student had been shot-gunning or using a beer bong. If you are drinking beer at a *normal* rate, most people fill up from the sheer volume, so they end up consuming far less total alcohol than when they are drinking mixed drinks or doing shots. The same holds true for wine and wine coolers, as these drinks are typically sipped and savored, not chugged.
  - **How do we know?** *Because it's the shot-takers who need our prescription antinausea medications and IV fluids!* The poster child for hangovers lies curled up on an exam room bed, reeling in between puking episodes and holding their pounding head, vowing, "I'm *never* again doing shots!"
- **Drink one full glass of water** after every alcoholic drink.
  - If not water, then any other noncaffeinated, nonalcoholic drink works. Party favorites include Topo Chico, La Croix, Sprite, vitamin waters, or sport drinks like Gatorade or Powerade.

- **Limit yourself to one alcoholic drink per hour** and decide your total limit *before* you start drinking.
- **Do not mix types of alcohol**
  - *Any combination in **any** order* increases your risk of hangover!
  - Fake news: "Liquor before beer, you're in the clear!"

What about HANGXIETY? Is it real?

Yes! Roughly 20 percent of college students experience hangover anxiety, a sometimes crippling "morning after" depressed or anxious mood after drinking to excess. This malady is known by many names: the Booze Blues, Hangover Blues, Drinking Depression, the "Saddies," or the currently popular "Hangxiety." Whatever you choose to call it, this frustrating condition makes more sense if we break it down by brain, body, and emotions.

BRAIN:
- Alcohol initially creates a joyful buzz as your brain is flooded with high levels of "happy" neurotransmitters, primarily dopamine and serotonin. Unfortunately, this leaves you with a relative deficit the next day, which can contribute to feeling sad or anxious.
- Meanwhile, although alcohol makes you sleepy, it disrupts the quality of your sleep, so your now sleep-deprived brain is adding to your anxiety.

BODY:
- As noted above, alcohol makes your heart race (from dehydration and vasodilation), drops your blood sugar (causing shakiness, nausea, and headache), and irritates your stomach lining and your liver (adding more nausea).
- All these symptoms signal your brain that you "feel" anxious, so you ARE anxious.

EMOTIONS:

- Lastly, there is often very valid anxiety over what you may or may not have done while judgment-impaired under the influence of alcohol, *especially if you have memory gaps*, and often surrounding the potential risks associated with physical intimacy.

What helps HANGXIETY?

Obviously, prevention is the best "cure," but the same things that help the physical pain of a hangover—hydration, complex carbohydrates, and pain relievers—will help ease many of the physical symptoms of anxiety. If your worry is more focused on physical intimacy issues, please do not wait—go get tested.

See Chapter 45, Sexually Transmitted Infections (Yes, It Happens to People like You) and Chapter 46, Date Rape and Sexual Assault.

TIPS:

- When drinking alcohol, **avoid caffeinated alcoholic beverages.**
  - You feel "fine" (not intoxicated) because caffeine makes you less sleepy with more energy, but your reaction times slow down and your judgment is impaired.

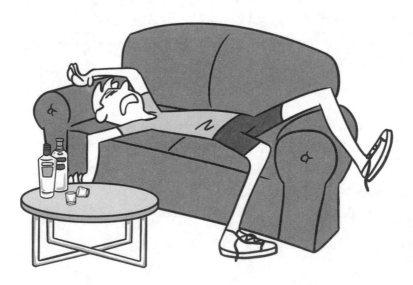

- O Caffeinated alcoholic drinks also increase impulsivity, which may encourage you to drink more than you intended, which then increases impulsivity even more . . . and so on.
- O ***Never mix alcohol with prescription pain killers***—this is deadly!
- O Coffee (or other caffeine source) does **not** reverse a hangover.
  - O Coffee actually makes hangovers worse by further dehydrating you.
- O When rehydrating for a hangover, **avoid using straws**—the extra air they add to your stomach will worsen your nausea.

Chapter 2
Other Bad Headaches (Migraines)

What If: I Get a Migraine?

Medical Name: Migraine Headache (with or without Aura)

What most likely happened:

You've had headaches before, but this was different. While you were studying, you developed blurry vision—hard to describe, but a portion of the paragraph seemed fuzzy or blacked out, forcing you to squint to decipher the words. Then the headache kicked in, and before long, the entire right side of your head was throbbing. Meanwhile, you didn't think it would be a good idea to take ibuprofen for fear it would further upset your increasingly nauseated stomach. Ultimately, all you could do was curl up in bed in a pitch-black, silent room for several hours till you fell asleep.

What's going on?

Many students use the word *migraine* to describe any severe headache, but migraine actually refers to a specific type of vascular headache that classically includes many of these elements:

- **Preheadache "Aura"** occurs within the first hour before/during your migraine, typically lasting five to twenty minutes before the headache begins (*note that not every migraine comes with an aura*):
    - Visual changes (most common symptoms):
        - Small sections of your vision obscured (white or black splotches)
        - Tunnel vision
        - Blurred vision
        - Shimmering lights or light flashes
    - Odd skin sensation (*paresthesias*) with tingling or numbness that often moves from your hands or arms to your face
    - Feeling of heaviness in your arms/legs or difficulty speaking
- **Pain on one side** of your head (occasionally on both); typically starts near temple and progresses back along that side of your head
- **Throbbing** (rather than the constant pressure of sinus or tension headaches)
- **Nausea** with or without vomiting
- Extreme **light or noise sensitivity**
- **Movement** makes headache worse

Treatment:
Mild-moderate headache:
- Over-the-Counter Nonsteroid Anti-Inflammatory Medications (OTC NSAIDs)
    - Ibuprofen (Advil)
    - OTC Naproxen (Aleve)—takes longer to kick in, but relief lasts longer without redosing
- Add to or substitute acetaminophen (Tylenol) for an NSAID above
- OTC Combo products with aspirin/acetaminophen/caffeine

Moderate-severe headache:
- **Prescription "Triptans":**

- **Stop migraine progression and abort the headache** by stimulating the neurotransmitter serotonin, reducing inflammation and constricting blood vessels
  - sumatriptan (Imitrex): injection, nasal spray, or tablets
  - rizatriptan (Maxalt): orally disintegrating tablets (ODT) or tablets
  - zolmitriptan (Zomig): nasal spray, ODT, or tablets
  - almotriptan (Axert) & eletriptan (Relpax): tablets
  - naratriptan (Amerge) & frovatriptan (Frova): tablets—slower onset but long-lasting
  - Triptans can be combined with NSAIDs like ibuprofen or naproxen
- **Ketorolac (Toradol):** injection (typically given in your arm)
  - Stronger NSAID; think of this as injectable super-ibuprofen, strong as a narcotic without the sedation
  - Injection is administered in the doctor's office/urgent care/ER
- **Preferred antinausea medications:**
  - Metoclopramide (Reglan)
  - Prochloperazine (Compazine)
- **Dihydroergotamine** (DHE nasal spray, muscle injection, or IV)
- **Infrequent "Others":** antiseizure or antipsychotic medications, steroids, and opioids

Head to your doctor if you have:
- The worst headache of your life.
- Prolonged nausea/vomiting.
- Fever.
- Headaches that interfere with school, work, or your social life.
- Headaches that don't respond to OTC pain relievers.
- Headaches that require any type of pain reliever more than 10 days per month.
  - At this frequency, you may be unintentionally causing "rebound" or "medication overuse" headaches.

Worst-case scenario:

Intractable migraines (*status migrainosus*) are rare (less than 1 percent of migraine sufferers) but severe migraine headaches last more than three days. Treatment requires hospitalization for IV hydration, steroids, and various combinations of pain control and anti-nausea medications.

Prevention:

- **Decaffeinate!** People who don't drink caffeine regularly can often very effectively use caffeine to stop a migraine—simply drink a coffee (or caffeinated beverage of choice) as soon as you feel warning signs of a migraine (changes in your vision, taste, or smell *before* your headache gets bad).
- **Exercise:** Daily aerobic exercise (ideally 30 minutes/day) raises your brain's serotonin levels and helps prevent migraines.
- **Stay Hydrated**: Dehydration often triggers migraines.
- **Good Nutrition:** Dropping blood sugar levels from skipping meals is another trigger, so always carry healthy snacks like high-protein granola bars or fruit and nuts in your backpack "just in case."
- **Sleep**: Inconsistent sleep/wake times aggravate migraines.
- **Identify Your Food and Drink Triggers** such as:
  - Alcohol
  - Chocolate
  - Aged cheeses
  - Diet drinks (or artificial sweeteners in anything, most commonly aspartame)
- **Prophylactic Migraine Therapy:** If you have more than three migraines/month, talk to your doctor about daily preventative medication choices.
- Daith piercings are ear cartilage piercings that some people believe may help decrease the severity or frequency of migraine headaches. I wish there were scientific data to support this, because I've anecdotally had several patients who failed Western medicine interventions and had improvement from daith

piercings, but we do not have evidenced-based support at this time. Note some people have worsening of their migraines after this piercing, and up to 30 percent have infections (as is the case with all ear cartilage piercings). Healing is long—eight to ten months—and it is recommended that you not sleep on the side of the piercing while it heals. *(See illustration of Daith Piercing on page 284.)*

TIPS:

○ Although stress can trigger headaches, **migraines often show up *after* stressors**, like the weekend after midterms, so be aware of this timing and avoid additional triggers and be sure to keep your ibuprofen/triptan in your backpack/purse.

○ Be proactive; if your weekend plans include triggers like alcohol, flashing lights, and loud pulsating music, *consider taking a preventative dose before you head out.*

○ **"Ice-Pick Headaches"** are a migraine variant: sudden, fleeting (usually one to three seconds) stabbing headaches, often recurring intermittently on the front or side of your head.

○ Just like *hormonal changes* during your period, *birth control pills may also trigger migraines*. Changing brand or type of pills often eliminates this unwanted side effect.

○ Many OTC combination products help migraines, typically combining caffeine and aspirin, Tylenol, or Advil. Another readily available option is taking acetaminophen (Tylenol) and ibuprofen (Advil) *together* along with a caffeinated beverage. These medications work through different pathways, so they are safe to take together at their recommended doses, and their combined effect is magnified.

○ EEGs (brain wave tracings) and neuroimaging with MRIs or CT scans are **rarely** indicated and usually unnecessary to diagnose migraines.

○ Migraines are a vascular phenomenon that can occur *with or without the headache*; if you have recurrent short-lived visual symptoms (especially if you have a family or personal history of migraines), talk to your doctor.

○ **Location, location, location!** Headaches fall in a spectrum with overlapping qualities, but where you hurt typically points to the cause:

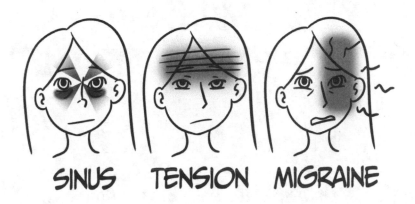

SINUS   TENSION   MIGRAINE

Chapter 3
I Hit My Head–
Do I Have a Concussion?

What If: I Hit My Head. Do I Have a Concussion?
Medical Name: Mild Traumatic Brain Injury (Mild TBI)

What most likely happened:

Scenario A: Playing intramural "noncontact" sports when a high-speed ball or another player directly hits your head, knocking your body to the ground and possibly knocking you briefly unconscious. Symptoms may begin immediately or a few hours after the injury.

Scenario B: Rental E-Scooter accidents. Same song, different verse—this time with your head hitting the pavement, a car, or a wall rather than a ball or person hitting you.

Scenario C: Party scene, doing shots . . . and that's all you remember. You wake up with a wicked headache, confusion, and possibly a bump on your head or scrapes and bruises on your hands/arms/legs that suggest you took a fall. This version typically includes backstory as friends text asking if you recovered from your fall or from "blacking out" last night.

What's going on?

A concussion is often described as a "brain bruise" that occurs from either a physical blow directly to the head or injuries elsewhere that transmit that force to the head, causing a **functional**—*not structural*—injury to the brain. The brain circuits are "shaken," but no bleeding or direct tissue damage occurs. Therefore, CT and MRI scans ***cannot*** determine whether you have a concussion. These scans may occasionally be used to look for additional injuries or complications, but they neither confirm nor deny the presence of a concussion, so do not automatically assume you will need one.

Concussions may create numerous temporary neurologic changes, most commonly:

- Headache
- Mood changes (anxiety, depression, irritability)
- Sleep disturbance (too much or too little)
- Nausea and/or vomiting
- Balance issues
- Light and/or noise sensitivity
- Difficulty focusing or "brain fogginess"

Treatment:

The answer is **complete brain rest** for twenty-four to forty-eight hours, then start low, go slow as you return to activities.

Brain Rest means: no screens, no texting, no reading, no listening to lectures. You need a quiet, darkened room where you can comfortably sleep. *The sooner and more completely you comply with complete brain rest, the sooner your brain will heal and you can return to activities.*

Note that **full academic return without worsening symptoms** should happen before you start back on exercise, sports, jobs, or clubs.

Basic Concussion Rehab

Each step should be twenty-four hours. Go back a step if symptoms worsen.

- **Step 1:** Complete cognitive rest for twenty-four to forty-eight hours.
- **Step 2:** Light routine physical activities (cooking, light house work) and trial of thirty-minute segments of cognitive tasks, such as reading/studying. When you are able to tolerate forty-five minutes of academic effort without worsening symptoms, you may return to class. (No work, no extracurricular, no sports yet.)
- **Step 3:** Full return to academics without worsening symptoms (headache, nausea, fatigue)
- **Step 4:** Light, nonimpact aerobic exercise (walking, exercise bike)
- **Step 5:** Moderate activity (treadmill, elliptical)
- **Step 6:** Return to work (low- or no-impact jobs) and nonphysical extracurriculars (meetings, etc.)
- **Step 7:** Sport-specific drills
- **Step 8:** Sport practice: noncontact
- **Step 9:** Sport practice with contact
- **Step 10:** Return to playing sports and full life activities

When to head to your doctor:

As a college student, if you have a head injury significant enough to lose consciousness or have any concussive symptoms, *please get checked out.* At a minimum, concussion inventory scales will give your doctor a baseline to reassess you if your symptoms persist. Professors are far more understanding when they see documentation that a doctor has placed you on short-term "complete brain rest" so you cannot prepare for a test, versus telling them the day of the exam that you couldn't study the last few days because you think you might have a concussion.

Worst-case scenario:

Concussions, by definition, are temporary neurologic changes, so the good news is that symptoms should resolve. Unfortunately, two "worst-case" scenarios exist:

- **Subdural Hematoma:** This potentially lethal injury comes from the brain being forcibly sloshed forward and backward rapidly, tearing tiny bridging veins above the brain and under the skull. Because bleeding is extremely slow, symptoms evolve over many days or even a couple of weeks. Instead of symptoms slowly improving, in this case symptoms show up and steadily worsen. If you feel basically okay after a significant head injury but then later in the week become confused or develop nausea, weakness, seizures, or a steadily worsening headache, now is the time for that CT scan to rule out this bleeding problem.

- **Repeat concussions** clearly have a detrimental effect on memory and mood, and research continues to evaluate the impact on cognition and long-term neurodegenerative diseases such as Alzheimer's and Chronic Traumatic Encephalopathy (CTE). Take-home message: the more concussions, the worse the outcome.

Prevention:
- **Helmets**—if you are riding a bike, motorcycle, or scooter, protect your brain!
- **Limit alcohol**—if you do drink, choose beer or wine, **not shots**.
- **Think!** You *know* standing on that wobbly chair or stool to hang posters or strings of lights is risky . . . but it's too much hassle to get a ladder, so you do it anyway. Or your phone or watch buzzes with a text while you're biking, scootering, or driving, and you reflexively "must" answer. Don't do it!!

TIPS:
- The biggest mistake college students make is **not actually resting** their brain. Taking a full day completely off studying, class, work, extracurricular activities, *and screens* will get you back to speed much faster than trying to cut back but continue your work load.
- **Concussion is a clinical diagnosis.** Most head injuries do **not** require a CT scan.
- **No driving** until cleared by your physician; your balance and reaction times are affected more than you realize.

- Bright lights frequently trigger headaches with concussions, so **wear sunglasses** if outside or in a brightly lit room.
- ***If you have a concussion, avoid ALCOHOL and any mind-altering substance (marijuana);*** *using these substances while your "brain bruise" is healing is like repeatedly hitting a recovering bruise on your arm.*

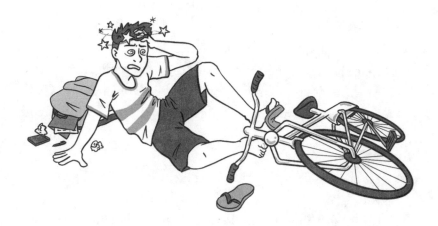

Chapter 4
I Can't Sleep!
Insomnia Issues

What If: I Can't Sleep?
Medical Name: Insomnia

What most likely happened:
Freshman September. Or a relationship ending. Or exams. The combination of extra noise from roommates/suitemates/dorm, unsettled sleep patterns, bedtime social media (and the FOMO that aggravates), academic adjustments, and other anxieties often blend together to create a downward spiral of fatigue and trouble concentrating, leading to poor grades . . . which cause more anxiety and more insomnia.

What's going on?
Obviously, numerous factors combine to mess up sleep, but typically:
- **Anxiety causes trouble falling asleep** (initial insomnia)
- **Depression** makes it **hard to stay asleep** (terminal insomnia); waking at "4:17 a.m." daily
- Stuffy nose, asthma, racing heart, medications, injuries, etc., may mess up your sleep

Treatment:
Behavioral Changes:

- Set a **consistent time** to wake up (at least within an hour window). Got a 9 a.m. class on MWF but don't start till 12:30 p.m. T/Th? *Different sleep and wake times each day don't jive with your body's internal clock.* Create a morning library study period or exercise time for yourself on T/Th that you treat as another mandatory 9 a.m. class so you get up and leave your dorm room the same time every day. Weekends? Maybe give yourself an extra hour, but you're honestly better off getting up at that same time and napping in the afternoon if you need it.

- **Daily aerobic exercise** (specifically thirty minutes of sustained heart rate elevation by walking, running, biking, elliptical machine, rowing, etc.) is a wonderful stress reducer, but because of the adrenaline it produces, make sure not to exercise within three hours of your normal bedtime.

- **Sleeping masks** are a great way to physically block out light in a shared space. Spend the extra few bucks for one that fits right, is easily washable, and is comfortable (usually around $15 to $20). Side notes: be sure to toss the mask in the wash once a week (to limit acne and skin irritation) and keep the mask on during the night—resist the temptation to check the time. If you can't cover your eyes, cover the clock/watch/iPhone. *Brains have the unwelcome superpower to wake you up at the exact time every night if you check the time.*

- **Block new noises** like snoring roommates, hallway traffic, or loud face-timing neighbors with a combination of comfortable ear plugs or extra white noise from a portable fan (even if you have A/C).

- **Guided meditation apps.** Try several and figure out what works best for you. Consider some of these top-ranked apps:
  - Headspace
  - Calm
  - 10% Happier

- The Mindfulness App
- Insight Timer
- **CBT-i Coach App**: This excellent free app utilizes effective cognitive behavioral therapy techniques specifically for insomnia (originally developed for military veterans).
- **Aromatherapy.** *Don't roll your eyes*—dorm rooms often **stink.** Mountains of dirty laundry, overflowing trash cans, and sweaty bedding don't add to your state of relaxation. While lighted candles are typically not allowed, plenty of other calming scents are—a spritz of Febreze, gelatin jars, wall-socket plug-in air fresheners, Pinterest-worthy herbal wreaths, electronic essential oil diffusers . . . Do **not**, however, start spraying perfumes/ colognes—that aggravates the smelly vortex. Consider tossing dryer sheets into drawers or hampers and commit to emptying the trash every few days and doing laundry at least twice per month.
- **Weighted blanket.** Picture a snuggly version of the radiation-blocking "aprons" that are draped over you during X-rays. Their comforting extra weight (fifteen to twenty pounds for adults) is calculated to feel like an extended hug, and clinical studies have shown anxiety reduction and sleep improvement.
  - Pricey ($40 to $150), but student discounts and coupons help. If you are texture sensitive (do you cut tags out of your shirts?), then purchase in a store (versus online) so you can touch and feel the material.
- **Foam mattress topper.** First-world issue, but college mattresses are not brilliant. Adding a couple inches of foam, egg-crate, or memory gel can dramatically improve comfort. Prices range from $15 to $150; most students find the $30–$50 range works great.
- **Decaffeinate.** Stop the afternoon Starbucks! Although significant individual variation exists for caffeine metabolism (based on two genes that control how quickly you break down caffeine), even

the people least sensitive to caffeine should not consume any for six hours before bedtime.

- **Decongestants** (e.g., Sudafed) are stimulants; use them in the morning only.
- **ADHD (Attention Deficit Hyperactivity Disorder) medications** are obviously stimulants, so be aware of how long your prescribed medication is active in your system, and then calculate the timing backward from bedtime for days where you may only have an afternoon or evening class.
- **Nicotine** is a stimulant. Stop vaping/smoking/dipping.
- **Alcohol** is a sedative, so yes, it may help you fall asleep; however, alcohol impairs your quality of sleep, often causing difficulty staying asleep.
- **Avoid screens** at least the last hour or two before bed. *Seriously!* Numerous studies have confirmed the detrimental effect of screen blue light on sleep cycles. Yes, you live on screens socially and academically, but simple modifications can make a difference.
  - Set study breaks to play games or peruse social media (rather than using this activity to relax at bedtime).
  - Save your book reading or off-screen math assignments for the end of your evening.
  - Move your shower time to immediately before bed, and take your time in the shower if no one is waiting. (Remember taking baths before bed as a child? Same concept.)
  - Use music or meditation apps as you wind down in bed.

Medications:
ALL medications are a distant second choice to behavioral modifications.
- Most OTC Sleep Aids contain antihistamine medications, typically diphenhydramine (Benadryl) as the "PM" ingredient. Aleve PM, Advil PM, Tylenol PM, ZZZQuil, etc.
- Unisom adds a different antihistamine, doxylamine succinate.

- Pros: Easily available, nonaddictive, may help short term
- Cons: Dry mouth, morning "hangover," constipation, effectiveness falls with continued use
- Nonantihistamine OTC sleep aids include:
  - Melatonin
    - Note that a higher dose does not make it more effective! In fact, if your insomnia is more of a delayed sleep phase disorder (your internal clock pushing back your sleep cycle by hours), the lowest doses of melatonin are often more effective.
    - Melatonin doesn't work immediately; optimal dosing ranges two to six hours before desired sleep time, and it may take several days to achieve the best effect in your body.
    - While melatonin requires a prescription in some other countries (Australia and some European countries), it is OTC in the United States. Note that nonprescription supplements do not have the same regulations as prescription drugs, so there can be greater variability in quality and efficacy between brands.
  - Valerian—may improve sleep quality over placebo, but studies are conflicting.
  - Tryptophan—an amino acid that converts to serotonin; again, mixed scientific results.

Note that American Academy of Sleep Medicine's evidence-based guidelines for insomnia treatment recommend against the use of diphenhydramine (Benadryl), melatonin, valerian, and tryptophan.

Prescription Sleep Medications:
No doubt you've seen ads for the "Z-drugs": Zolpidem (Ambien), esZopiclone (Lunesta) or Zaleplon (Sonata); these are all hypnotic medications designed to be less-addictive options for the treatment of

insomnia, as compared to benzodiazepines like alprazolam (Xanax) and diazepam (Valium), which are clearly addictive. Unfortunately, turns out that the "Z-drugs" can cause tolerance (need more of the drug for the same effect), dependence (without the drug you have withdrawal symptoms), and even addiction (overwhelming desire to take the drug). Additionally, mixing these drugs with alcohol is particularly dangerous, as the combination dramatically suppresses your drive to breathe. For these reasons, physicians no longer prescribe these medications long-term, but your doctor may consider a very limited prescription (less than a week) if your insomnia has been resistant to all other interventions.

Other nonaddictive classes of prescription medications such as antihistamines, seizure medications, and antidepressants may also be used for their sedating side effects.

Head to your doctor if:
You've tried the nonmedicinal behavioral changes first, but your insomnia persists more than a week. *Please don't wait until your grades are tanked!* Daytime sleepiness (falling asleep in class), inability to concentrate enough to effectively study, or out-of-control emotions should all send you directly to the doctor.

Worst-case scenario:
The vast majority of college student insomnia is situational (physical, environmental, or emotional), so the most common worst case is treatment with therapy and/or medications for underlying depression or anxiety. Numerous other medical conditions may aggravate or cause insomnia, most commonly seasonal allergies, infections, injuries, asthma, heartburn/reflux, and thyroid disorders, obviously requiring different treatment. Last, other sleep disorders like restless legs syndrome, sleep apnea, and narcolepsy may initially show up during college years.

Prevention:

- Healthy sleep hygiene:
    - Consistent sleep/wake times
    - Control environment (light, noise, odors, physical comfort)
- Consistent daily aerobic exercise
- Reduce stressors
- Limit stimulants
- Limit alcohol

TIPS:

- If academic stress is the primary source of your anxiety and subsequent insomnia, do not suffer in silence or wait till you "have" to talk to your professor. **Go to tutoring!** Almost everyone is initially overwhelmed by the volume and intensity of college courses, *especially if you got in to your "dream" school.*
- Learning to utilize study partners or groups, attending tutoring sessions, and discovering new interactive memorization techniques will help dramatically. Locking yourself in a room "until I finish," skipping fun activities as you try to force-feed

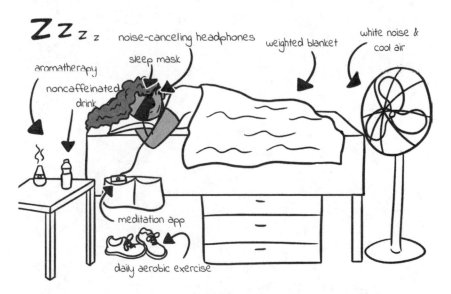

ZZz z noise-canceling headphones weighted blanket white noise & cool air

sleep mask

aromatherapy

noncaffeinated drink

meditation app

daily aerobic exercise

yourself the information, will be minimally productive, if at all. Alternating study locations, prioritizing sleep, and taking practice tests will improve your grades. All-nighters do not.

o **FOMO is quicksand**. When **all** your friends at other universities look like they are having way more fun than you are . . . *look at your own posts* and realize you are likely projecting the same image to them.

o Sliding mattress topper messing up your sleep? Make sure you have the right size (twin toppers slide on twin XL mattresses). Still sliding? Get a skid-resistant grip pad (around $15) like Gorilla Grip, SensorPedic, or Secure Grip.

Chapter 5
Test Anxiety

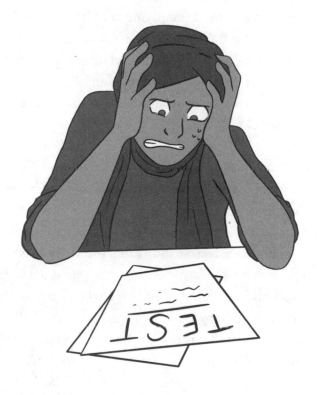

What If: I Get Awful Test Anxiety?

Medical name: Social Phobia

What most likely happened:

Your first general chemistry test blew you out of the water, despite the fact that you were a straight-A, top-10 percent student in high school. Now even weekly quizzes make your heart pound like it's trying to leap out of your chest while dripping sweat soaks your shirt. At times, your lips and fingertips start tingling, and then your brain goes into a panic and you cannot concentrate enough to do well on your quiz, turning your premed dreams into college nightmares.

What's going on?

Mental anxiety triggers our body's fight-or-flight reaction, *whether or not the fears are realistic.* The body prepares to run by revving up the heart rate and dumping excess weight (emptying your bowels and bladder). The total anxiety response also includes shortness of breath, actual or perceived muscle shaking, sweating, upset stomach, and brain fogginess that includes difficulty concentrating, fear, and "blanking out."

NOTE: Up to 20 percent of students suffer from intense test anxiety. You are not alone!

Treatment:

The good news is that you have both behavioral and medicinal options to help reduce or eliminate test anxiety.

- **Cognitive behavioral therapy (CBT)**—either individual or group—is **highly effective** in treating social phobias. This "talk therapy" helps people recognize how they are unconsciously magnifying and catastrophizing potential negative outcomes that trigger the physical anxiety responses.
  - Please note CBT is not "lie on a couch and tell me why you hate your mother" therapy! CBT is more like a study skills course that teaches you tools to replace knee-jerk emotional responses with thoughtful, productive solutions.
- **Breathing exercises**—many variations exist, but an easy start is to take one full minute to focus on your breathing before you enter the testing room, and again just before you start the exam or give your talk. Breathe in for a slow count of four and then breathe out for a slow count of ten. Repeat this sequence three or four times till you feel your body relaxing.

- **Study skills training**—obviously, if your test anxiety is coming from poor preparation, the primary answer is learning more effective study habits.
- **Medications**—
  - The most common prescription medication used is actually a blood pressure medication (a beta-blocker called metoprolol) that is used in low doses primarily for the side effect of *slowing the heart rate and reducing tremors*.
  - Interestingly, when the physical sensations of racing heart and tremor are stopped, the brain "hears" that the body is not stressed, and frequently this is enough to lower the test anxiety down to an expected, manageable level. *This type of medication is not addictive.*
  - Other social phobias such as fear of flying may be medically managed with sedatives called benzodiazepines, such as alprazolam (brand name Xanax). Note that these medications are very addictive, often misused, and sedating, so they are NOT a good option for test anxiety.

Head to your doctor if:
- You need help—please do **not** wait for finals or even midterms! Know that campus physicians treat this very frequently, and we are happy to see you as soon as you are concerned.
- You realistically assess whether your anxiety is from lack of effective preparation versus being fully prepared but overly anxious. If you are acing practice tests and homework but blanking out on actual exams, medication may help dramatically.
- Behavioral interventions should ideally be tried before considering medication, but often we initiate both at the same time.

Worst-case scenario:

Untreated test anxiety can lead to a down-spiraling nightmare. "Bombing" one test leads to more anxiety on the second, because now you desperately need to raise your grade from the first test. That heightened anxiety worsens your symptoms, likely causing a worse grade on the next test and so on, until your entire course's grade is sunk for the semester or you begin having test anxiety in other classes, as well.

Prevention:

- **Time management** is the biggest challenge for most college freshmen, so many schools have Student Success Programs that offer free counseling that specifically teach students how to create study schedules.
- *If you never had to work hard to make good grades in high school, you may actually need to learn basic study techniques—* don't let your ego keep you from seeking help.
  - Start with your university's website and search "study skills" or "test anxiety." Odds are good you can find free workshops and classes in addition to online basics that can dramatically improve how effectively and efficiently you study and prepare for exams.
- **Study skills include strategies for both solo and effective group study:**
  - Learning to convert ten-minute time pockets (otherwise wasted on social media perusal or games) into quick study sessions of self-created flash cards or online quizzes.
  - Changing study locations and times to optimize mental energy.
  - Reviewing concepts out loud (alone or, better, with a partner).
  - Creating acronyms or "chaining" rather than rote memorization.
  - Finding and taking multiple practice tests.
  - Learning which review sessions are most helpful (*possibly not your section's TA or prof*).
  - Test strategies like "brain dumps"—learning to quickly scribble down formulas or names you might forget in the first minute of a test.

- Your university's student success program is the very best place to start (free and convenient, with local knowledge), but know there are private tutorial businesses and numerous one-on-one tutorials online from professors at other universities teaching the same topics. (Prices range from $30 to $60 an hour.) If you don't connect with one program or instructor, keep looking! Especially when you are having trouble with specific concepts in a course, spending an hour or two with a private tutor may be a grade changer.
- **Arrive early** for your event to avoid the extra anxiety that comes from rushing and fear of arriving late.
- Greatly **reduce or, preferably, eliminate caffeine** and other stimulants (like decongestants) for at least several days before your exam. Caffeine both aggravates the physical symptoms directly and impairs the quality of your sleep, which subsequently worsens symptoms.
- **Eat** a meal or at least a snack that contains some fat or protein within two hours before your event. Primarily carbohydrate snacks or meals, even if healthy (like fruit, cereal, or a pasta and veggie meal), can aggravate physical symptoms by causing a blood sugar crash.
  - Example: Have some nuts or peanut butter along with apple slices, rather than eating an apple by itself.
- **Exercise**—increase your heart rate for a sustained twenty to thirty minutes daily in your aerobic activity of choice; walking is fine, but really push the speed. Strolling will get you mood-elevating sunshine with Vitamin D, but to most effectively reduce stress, you want to put out enough effort to break a sweat.

TIPS:

○ If you are prescribed an as-needed test anxiety medication, take it for the first time when you have a minor quiz that you are nervous about but not freaking out over. This should give you a chance to assess any potential side effects plus hopefully give you a positive experience to boost your confidence.

○ Study schedules start with literally writing out your class schedule in an hourly week-long template, but add in meals, meetings, events, and specific study time frames and locations. Getting a visual plan is critical to avoiding last-minute panic, cramming, and all-nighters (which all increase test anxiety and decrease performance).

○ Most universities have their own study tips and schedule templates that you can easily download and print. Search "academic resources" on the main university website and look for sections such as "study strategies" or "academic success" tips. Some may require logging in as a student for access, though others, such as Baylor's, Texas A&M's, and LMU's, are publicly available.

	Mon	Tues	Wed	Thurs	Fri	Sat	Sun
8am							
9am		Calculus ↓		Calculus ↓			Work Front Desk
10am	Chem 101		Chem 101		Chem 101	Library	(Bring HW)
11am							↓
12pm	Spanish 301	Lunch	Spanish 301	Lunch	Spanish 301		
1pm	Lunch	Intro Econ	Lunch	Intro Econ	Lunch	Lunch	Lunch
2pm	Chem Lab	↓		↓			
3pm			Library			State vs Tech Tailgate	
4pm	↓	Spin class		Spin class		& Football	
5pm			↓				Church
6pm	Dinner	Dinner	Dinner	Dinner	Dinner		Dinner w/ Young Life
7pm	Calc HW	Work Front Desk			Homework in dorm room or Lounge		
8pm	Study group	(Bring HW)	Homework in dorm Study Lounge	LAB Tutorial			
9pm	Madrigal Singers	↓					
10pm							
11pm							
12am							

Chapter 6
Fear of Public Speaking and Classroom Anxiety

What If: I Get Anxiety with Public Speaking?
Medical name: Social Phobia or Glossophobia

What most likely happened:
This semester, you have a major individual presentation in your business class that counts for 20 percent of your total grade. The mere thought of standing up and speaking in front of a large group is making your hands sweat, heart race, chest tighten up, and guts cramp up. How will you be able to perform effectively?

OR

In your seminar-style classes, a significant portion of your grade is class participation. Though you never had issues in high school, now you are suddenly afraid that you might look dumb compared to your peers, which makes you hesitant to raise your hand and comment or ask questions.

What's going on?
Just like with test anxiety, any type of mental anxiety triggers our body's fight-or-flight reaction, *whether or not the fears are realistic*. The body prepares to run by revving up the heart rate and dumping excess weight

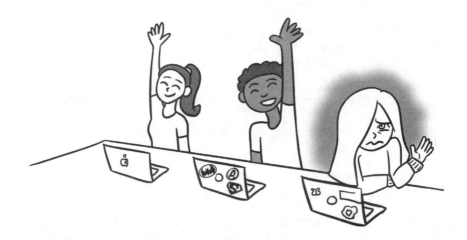

(emptying your bowels and bladder). The total anxiety response includes shortness of breath, actual or perceived muscle shaking, sweating, upset stomach, and brain fogginess that includes difficulty concentrating, fear, and even "blanking out."

Fear of public speaking is the single most common phobia, with prevalence estimates ranging from 30 percent up to 75 percent of the population. A 2017 study focusing on college students revealed that 63.9 percent of students reported fear of public speaking, and 89.3 percent wanted their education to include classes to improve this skill. Comedian Jerry Seinfeld frequently jokes that people would rather be in the coffin than giving a eulogy at funerals (*since many people fear public speaking more than they fear death*), and he's right—you are not alone with this fear!

Treatment:

The good news is that you have both behavioral and medicinal options to help reduce or eliminate your public speaking anxiety.

- **Cognitive behavioral therapy (CBT)**—either individual or group—is highly effective in treating social phobias, including glossophobia. This "talk therapy" helps people recognize how they are unconsciously magnifying and catastrophizing potential negative outcomes, which triggers the physical anxiety responses.

- **Breathing exercises**—Many variations exist, but an easy start is to take one full minute to focus on your breathing before you stand up to give your talk. Breathe in for a slow count of four and then breathe out for a slow count of ten. Repeat this sequence three or four times till you feel your body relaxing. If you are in a class situation where multiple students are presenting before you go up, practice this exercise each time a new speaker begins their talk.

- **Medications**—
  - The most common medication prescribed for fear of public speaking is actually a blood pressure medication (a beta-blocker called metoprolol) that is used in low doses primarily for the side effect of ***slowing the heart rate and reducing tremors***. This medication can be taken as needed, rather than taken daily for prevention.
  - Interestingly, when the physical sensations of racing heart and tremor are stopped, the brain "hears" that the body is not stressed, and frequently this is enough to lower your fear of public speaking down to an expected, manageable level. Note that this type of medication is **not** addictive.
  - Other social phobias such as fear of flying may be medically managed with sedatives called benzodiazepines, such as alprazolam (brand name Xanax). However, this class of medications is **very** addictive, often misused, and too sedating, so it is not a good option for public speaking anxiety.

- **Regular Aerobic Exercise** has been shown to be an effective adjunctive treatment for anxiety, especially when combined with group CBT.

Head to your doctor if:

- Your anxiety is keeping you from participating in seminars or small class discussions beyond the first week or two of the semester.

- You have even one class with a huge (grade-weighted) presentation you are worried about. Please do **not** wait till the week of your presentation to seek help! Know that campus physicians treat this very frequently, and we are happy to see you as soon as you are concerned.
- You realistically assess whether your anxiety is lack of effective preparation versus being fully prepared, but overly anxious. *(This seems obvious, but it is important to recognize that medications alone will not improve your presentations if the actual problem is that you have not yet learned and developed the skills to prepare an effective talk.)*
- Behavioral interventions should ideally be tried before considering medication, but often we initiate both at the same time.

Worst-case scenario:

Untreated public speaking anxiety can lead to a down-spiraling situation. If you are too anxious to speak effectively to participate in class or give a presentation, then the next time you may become more anxious because you desperately need to raise your grade, so your anxiety is worse, and so on . . . until you have dug an enormous academic hole.

Prevention:

- Practice, practice, practice—in front of a mirror or, if you can, in front of a friend. Say the entire speech **out loud**—no short cuts—and practice at least once fully dressed and groomed as you will be for the presentation.
  - Media experts recommend "dressing for success" even when doing radio shows from home phones, because you feel more prepared.
  - If it's possible to actually practice in the empty classroom where you will be giving your talk, go there and **do it**! Nothing gives confidence like literally having stood at that podium before. Feel weird doing that alone? Ask a classmate if they want to meet in the room the night before

and take turns giving the speech to each other. If the room is locked/not available, at least visualize that setting while you rehearse.

- Use your phone to video yourself so you can see what is effective and what needs improvement.
- If possible, limit words on your slides—if **you** are reading from your visual aid, *so is the audience*, and they will not be engaged. **Images > Words**!
- Know your topic—*really know it*, don't simply memorize a speech. If you don't know it well enough to answer questions, you are not ready yet.

TIPS:
- Arrive early for your event to avoid the extra anxiety that comes from rushing and the fear of arriving late.
- Greatly reduce or preferably eliminate caffeine and other stimulants (like decongestants) for a couple of days before your speech. Caffeine both aggravates the physical symptoms directly and impairs the quality of your sleep, which subsequently worsens symptoms.
- Eat a meal or at least a snack that contains some fat or protein an hour or two before your speech. Primarily carbohydrate snacks or meals, even if healthy (like fruit, cereal, or a pasta and veggie meal), can aggravate physical symptoms by causing a blood sugar crash.
  - Add nuts, peanut butter, hummus, or cheese along with apple slices, rather than eating an apple by itself.

Chapter 7
Homesickness, Anxiety, and Depression

What If: I'm Homesick, Anxious, or Depressed?
Medical Name: Adjustment Disorder with Anxious/Depressed Mood

What most likely happened:
Transitions are hard, and for most college freshmen, this is the greatest transition of their lives. You may have been the smartest or most popular student before, but perhaps in the first month you've already bombed a test and been rejected by the top group you wanted to join, leaving you feeling unintelligent and anonymous. Or perhaps high school was socially awful, and you kept hearing how great college would be . . . but it's not yet. Or maybe you have been sick, ended a relationship, or suffered some type of loss or trauma. Or maybe it's financial stress. Or you have a family history of depression/anxiety and your brain chemistry is working against you. Meanwhile, Snapchat, Instagram, TikTok, and Facebook confirm everyone else you know is having a fabulous time, making you feel even more sad and isolated.

What's going on?

Anxiety and depression are painfully common during college years. Data from the American College Health Association National College Health Assessment in Spring 2023 reveals that, within the last year, 74.1% of students reported moderate to severe psychological distress, 50.8% had significant lonliness, 20% of students treated for depression, 45% of students felt so depressed it was difficult to function, 65.7% felt overwhelming anxiety, 28% were at risk for suicide (had a positive suicide screening test), 11% intentionally harmed themselves, and 2.3% attempted suicide.

Everyone experiences emotional ups and downs, but what is "too much"?

If your emotions are keeping you from doing what you want to do or what you should be doing, that's too much.

Ask yourself:

- Is stress, emotional inertia, or physical fatigue making you avoid or skip social gatherings, class, meetings, meals, or work?
- Are you not sleeping or, conversely, sleeping way too much?
- Are you self-medicating with food, alcohol, pot, or other drugs?
- Do you have enough energy for routine hygiene (showering, changing clothes)?
- Are you unable to concentrate enough to study and complete assignments?
- Are you having panic attacks or persistent worry about future panic attacks?
- Are you skipping class when there is an assignment due, a quiz, or a test you aren't ready for (and perhaps even e-mailing the professor you were sick)?
- Do you feel everyone is constantly judging you (even in common situations like meals)?
- Do you feel hopeless, helpless, overwhelmed, worthless, numb, persistently sad, or apathetic?
- Are you having thoughts of harming yourself?

If the answer is YES to any of these questions, it's time to see your doctor or a counselor.

Additionally, if your friend, classmate, or roommate is showing any of these signs, please encourage them to seek help. Better yet, *offer to walk with them over to the health center* AND tell someone—an RA, professor, counselor, or doctor. If you don't feel comfortable reaching out in person, then **go online to your campus health services and email them.** Many universities also have anonymous "behavior concerns advice lines" where mental health professionals can give you advice on how best to help your friend, plus most will reach out directly to that student.

The "988 Suicide & Crisis Lifeline" is now available in the United States and staffed 24/7 to offer free and confidential support. You can call or text "988" or go online to https://988lifeline.org and chat with a counselor at any time. They will listen and offer prevention and crisis resources for you or your loved one.

"988" Is our "911" for mental health!

Treatment:

Rarely is a single cause creating your anxiety or depression, so treatment is multifaceted:

- **Medical evaluation**: A physical exam +/- blood tests can help discover any physiologic or infectious problems aggravating your symptoms, especially with fatigue and low energy. Common findings include:
  - Mononucleosis
  - Anemia from heavy periods or a low meat or vegetarian diet
  - High or low thyroid hormone levels
  - Low Vitamin D levels
- **Health Habits:** Have you maximized behavioral changes?
  - Consistent sleep patterns (at least waking up the same time every day)

- Nutrition (are you skipping meals or severely lacking enough vegetables/fruit?)
- Exercise—thirty minutes of sustained aerobic activity each day (anything that raises your heart rate works) improves your brain neurotransmitters (serotonin, norepinephrine, and dopamine) comparable to a low-dose antidepressant medication.
- Alcohol, nicotine, and pot may seem to offer immediate "relief" but actually aggravate anxiety and depression.
- **Therapy:** College Health Centers typically offer an array of truly helpful advice, both group skills and individual therapy.
  - **Cognitive Behavioral Therapy (CBT)** is not lying on a couch talking about your mother, nor simply someone repeatedly asking, "How do you feel about that?" CBT involves insightful questions and discussions that help people recognize how they are unconsciously magnifying and using a catastrophic lens to view potential negative outcomes. CBT is typically short-term, goal-directed, and focuses on awareness with subsequent control and redirection of knee-jerk emotional reactions.
- **Student Services**: If your stress has affected your grades or class attendance, treatment may include meeting with your dean or advisor about a medical request to late-drop one class. If your primary stress is academic, see what your school offers:
  - Strengths assessment and career counseling
  - Individual or group tutoring
  - Peer academic coaching
  - Public speaking or time-management workshops
- **Medications:** Prescription medications are not mandatory but often provide tremendous relief. Many choices are available; your doctor can discuss benefits and side effects.

Homesickness: It may surprise you that homesickness is not limited to those students traveling far from home—we see it all the time (often worse!)

in students who have moved into a dorm from across town. This heartache is more about missing the "familiar"—your private bedroom and/or bathroom, home-cooked meals, established friend groups and routines, and yes, your family and beloved pets. Treatment focuses on establishing new roots and limiting time spent connecting with "home."

- Stop going home on weekends and limit your social media browsing.
- Don't be afraid to "third wheel" if your significant other is long-distance.
- Find a list of ten "must-do" things unique to your campus or town and do one each week.
- Look for someone else who feels the same way (there will be many!) but don't only commiserate: make plans and go to new events/locations, if only to study together.
- If you're in a dorm, talk to your RA! They're required to attend many dorm and school functions and happy to bring you along.

Worst-case scenario:

Not asking for help! You've worked far too hard to be in this college or university to suffer in silence or spiral down into a cycle of withdrawal or academic disaster. These issues are extremely common, and college/university health services want to help—*that's why we are here!*

Prevention:

- **Gratitude journals** have been repeatedly proven to improve well-being and reduce depression. Harvard Medical School Professor Dr. Sanjiv Chopra believes practicing gratitude on a daily basis (*through activities such as journaling*) is critical for our mental and physical health. Dr. Chopra frequently shares the anonymous quote: "If you don't know the language of gratitude, you'll never be on speaking terms with happiness." Practically speaking, how can you learn this as a busy and possibly overwhelmed college student?
  - **Each day, write down three specific things** you appreciate. Better to say, "I'm grateful my suitemates finally cleaned the

shower," than "I'm grateful for my suitemates." ***Consider who or what inspired you, or simply what comforts you that you might take for granted.*** Perhaps you can be grateful that you own more clothes than will fit inside your dorm closet, or that you have healthy legs to carry you across campus. Simply look around and challenge yourself to appreciate something different each day, both the ordinary and the extraordinary.

- If a hand-written journal doesn't appeal to you, consider creating a strictly ***private*** **Instagram account** where each day you post a quick pic and list at least one thing you are grateful for that day—a fall leaf, a new friend, an interesting class, clean socks, making it to your classes on time. The main rule is that this account is only for you, **not** for others to see and "like"—simply a **private visual diary, no followers**. Later, on your rough days, you'll have a beautiful quick reminder to scan about what's been good this year.

- **Health Habits** listed above, especially ***exercise!*** It bears repeating: thirty minutes every day. Sign up for at least one weekly group exercise activity (Zumba, yoga, hip-hop, ballroom dance, Frisbee golf, whatever!)

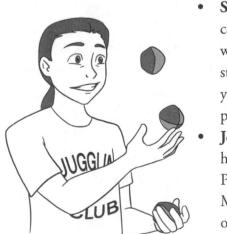

- **Socialize**. Yes, even if you are introverted, commit to at least one meal per week with another person and find places to study outside your dorm room; even if you sit at a table alone, there is benefit to physically being around others.

- **Join a Club**: Belonging to **any** group helps, from intramural sports to Harry Potter Quidditch, to Animation, Foodie, Movie, Religious, Service Organizations, or even a Juggling Club!

- **Volunteer**: Anywhere that interests you! Social justice opportunities abound on virtually every campus. Look for teams making sandwiches for people experiencing homelessness, mentoring at-risk grade school kids, or teaching English as a second language (ESL).

- **Lead:** This may seem counterintuitive, but leadership positions for dorm life (Residence Hall Associations), smaller clubs, and even student government often initially go unfilled—especially freshmen spots. Offering to serve an organization as a support position on their exec board is a great way to connect with like-minded students (and, in a good way, forces you to attend regular meetings).

- **Work:** Look for a low-stress part-time job on campus for a few hours per week (typically six hours is the maximum recommended). Universities have built-in job turnover and seem to always need more students to help set up events (placing chairs and tables), work info, and lost and found desks, etc. Many of the desk jobs are "slow" enough that you may be allowed to do homework while waiting for the phone to ring or customers to walk up.

TIPS:

o No matter how compassionate and responsible you are, the typical young college student is not a trained mental health provider, meaning you are not fully equipped to advise and help others who may be in crisis. Isn't this obvious? No! We often see students emotionally beating themselves up not because of their own situation, but over their roommate's or friend's or classmate's problems (*which becomes their problems because they are spending countless hours and energy trying to help*). While reaching out to others is important and admirable, know that **you are NOT fully responsible for anyone else's well-being**. Depressed friends may beg you not to tell anyone about their problems because they only want to vent to you. That's fine for minor issues, but *when you are* *worried about someone harming themselves,* do not wait to involve a medical professional.

○ **Antianxiety/antidepressant medications kick in slowly**—my mantra is the first week you get side effects (slight dizziness, nausea, or sleep disturbance), second week side effects improve, third week your friends see a difference, and fourth week you wonder why you didn't start this medication months ago. While some people have rapid improvement with anxiety symptoms (placebo? maybe, but good news regardless), be patient if you don't see dramatic changes the first few weeks.

○ **Light box therapy** (*literally a bright, full-spectrum light source*) may be helpful if your symptoms are worse in the winter (fewer hours of daylight), especially if you moved from the Sunbelt to a much cloudier, overcast climate in the northwestern or northeastern United States.

○ **Animal lover?** Look for some **"pet therapy"**! Many universities have therapy dogs and "pet-a-puppy" sessions, but most random dog owners are also happy to share some canine love (ask first, please). Students often miss their pets more than their families; people can connect with apps like FaceTime, but most animals aren't interested in no-smell technology.

○ **Social media-induced FOMO (Fear of Missing Out) is** *quicksand*. If looking at social media is making you feel bad, stop, or at least intensely limit looking at it. Literally set a timer and give yourself only ten minutes a day to scan it (preferably not right before going to sleep).

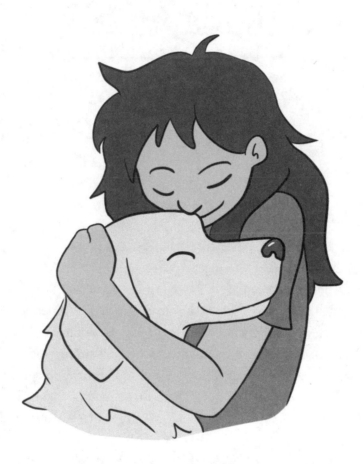

Chapter 8
Stimulants 101 (ADHD Meds, Risks, and Mistakes)

What If: I Take ADHD Medications?

Approximately 11 percent of current college students are diagnosed with Attention Deficit Hyperactivity Disorder, most of whom are treated with controlled substance prescription stimulants such as Adderall, Vyvanse, or Ritalin. Other students choose to "borrow" or purchase these pills to enhance their focus and keep them awake while cramming for an exam or writing a paper. Some students seek out these medications to suppress their appetites and lose weight. If you take prescribed ADHD meds or are considering "trying" them unprescribed, here are a few **TIPS** you should know:

- **Purchasing or selling these pills is a FELONY.**
  - Stimulants like ADHD medications are tightly regulated by the Drug Enforcement Agency. *Are you likely to get caught?* Perhaps not, but one felony charge IS guaranteed to ruin your life, and you never know when baby-faced campus police or DEA agents are undercover. Most college students picture drug dealers as stereotypical shady characters

in dark alleys. Readjust your lens to recognize the most common campus version: your well-meaning frat brother or sorority sister, that super sweet suite-mate or roommate, or even that overly brilliant classmate offering you "a little something" to get through pledge week, midterms, or a group project. What you learned in kindergarten still works: **just say no.**

- **ALWAYS keep your prescription medications in a locked box**, so none of your roommates or friends will be tempted to try one.
- **Use a medication reminder app or other system** (like a weekly pill box) to be sure you are accurately taking your medication. While forgetting to take your pills is a nuisance that may leave you feeling mentally sluggish or fatigued, **accidentally taking double your dose is dangerous**—especially if you are on a higher dose (like 40 to 60mg Vyvanse).
  - **Seriously? Yes.** Even "only" twice the stimulant will make your heart race and pound like crazy, with skipped beats and fast, irregular rhythms that can make you pass out or even cause a heart attack.
  - Your nervous system will be on overload, with intense tremors, headache, and possible hallucinations or confusion.
  - This scenario occurs most often around midterms or finals, when students' schedules are disrupted from the norm.
    - "I was up studying all night and then took my ADHD medication before heading to my 8:00 a.m. exam. Afterward, I went back to my dorm and crashed for a couple hours, and when I got up to start studying for my next class, I took another dose to help wake me up. Twenty minutes later, I got super shaky, started feeling nauseated, and now my heart's racing and doing flip-flops in my chest and I'm terrified that I could have a heart attack or something!"

- The challenging factor is that these medications stay in your system for six to eight hours, so although you may not "feel" anything from your dose of four or five hours ago, the drug is there, and adding in another dose can send your levels through the roof.

- **ADHD Meds will not magically improve your grades**.
  - Will taking a stimulant help you focus if you do not have ADHD?
    - Yes, it likely will—it's speed. Caffeine does the same.
    - In non-ADHD people, prescription stimulants do increase sustained focus attention but also increase distractibility, because these drugs increase impulsivity.
  - Will it help your grade (if you don't have ADHD)? Unlikely.
    - Broad studies looking at students taking prescription ADHD meds (whether or not they are diagnosed with ADHD) do not show improved GPAs, possibly because while the increased focus may help with immediate rote learning and memorization, the benefits extend to neither complex memory nor cognitive flexibility (which is standard fare for college exams).
    - "All-nighters" have been proven time and time again to be less helpful to your test grade than getting adequate sleep with less studying the night before.

- **What about caffeine?**
  - Caffeine is also a stimulant. (Ask your parents about NoDoz, the frequently abused caffeine source of choice by college students in the eighties, pre-Starbucks and Red Bull.) Any caffeine source—a pill, a cup of coffee, an "energy shot" like 5-Hour Energy or an energy drink like Red Bull—will have similar (if not quite as effective) temporary benefits.

- Caffeine in doses of 75 mg to 400mg (the max recommended daily dose is 400 mg) can temporarily increase focus, alertness, and simple memory tasks.
- For the biochemistry majors: Caffeine works in the brain by blocking adenosine receptors and secondarily increasing epinephrine (adrenaline) and dopamine.
- Caffeine also has **negative** side effects: insomnia,* heartburn, feeling jittery or anxious, racing heart, palpitations, and, of course, withdrawal headaches once you are drinking enough daily to become physically dependent. High doses of caffeine, especially when combined with ADHD meds, magnify these negative side effects—often sending students to the ER with chest pain, racing and irregular heart rhythms, panic attacks, and even seizures. (*Note that you may be able to fall asleep without difficulty, but if caffeine is still in your system, you are not getting that deep, restful sleep that fully rejuvenates our brains.)
- Take-home message: If you are prescribed ADHD medications, limit (or omit) caffeinated beverages from your daily routine. One stimulant source is enough.

ADHD Meds and Alcohol

"Pre-Gaming" with ADHD medications before going out drinking is an incredibly dangerous trend discovered by young people on these medications who found they could "hold their liquor" better if they happened to drink while the medicine was still in their system. Because ADHD medications keep the mind alert, a brain stimulated by them does not immediately react to the sedating qualities of alcohol.

- You have one drink; you feel perfectly fine.
- Take another, nothing.
- And another, and perhaps one or two more (especially if doing shots and therefore drinking quickly). But *then*, you zoom from feeling normal to buzzed to totally drunk, possibly blacking out.

- Even if you don't pass out, consider that even though you were not "feeling" the alcohol hit you, the alcohol in your blood was still rising, irritating your stomach lining and liver, plus slowing your reflexes (which includes your gag reflex).
- Fast-forward to intense nausea and vomiting . . . *and you can choke on that vomit.* Picture when you drink a sip of water and a drop or two "go down the wrong pipe," sending you into violent coughs to clear that water from your lungs, because the water went into your air pipe instead of your food pipe. Now imagine yourself nearly or fully passed out, and up comes your stomach contents and you have no gag reflex to keep that liquid from spilling into your air pipe . . . and you can lethally choke.

Bottom line: Taking prescribed ADHD medications early in the morning and then having an alcoholic drink or two in the evening adds minimal significant risk, but drinking alcohol while your ADHD medication is still active in your system (eight to fourteen hours, depending on the specific medication) is ***dangerous***.

Chapter 9
Passed Out: Alcohol Poisoning

What If: Someone Passes Out after Drinking Alcohol?
Medical Name: Alcohol toxicity

What most likely happened:
Freshman year, you're at a frat party with your pledge brothers, pounding vodka shots. No one wants to seem "weak" and not be able to handle their liquor, so everyone is drinking way more than they should. Your best friend was staggering around, slurring his words, barely able to keep his eyes open and hold his head upright, and now you spy him passed out on the couch. The upperclassmen tell you to move him to a bed and use the Bacchus Maneuver, but honestly, you're pretty drunk, scared, and don't really know what to do.

What's going on?
Alcohol poisoning goes far beyond puking.

Here's the **Blood Alcohol Concentration (BAC) breakdown**:

- When BAC reaches 0.12 (five drinks if you weigh 150 pounds), there is usually enough nausea to induce vomiting.

- When BAC hits 0.2 (approximately eight drinks if you weigh 150 pounds), most people will "black out" or "brown out," meaning they will have memory loss for all or some of what happened while they were drinking.
- When BAC crosses 0.3 (twelve drinks at 150 pounds), most people pass out (lose consciousness).
- If BAC reaches or exceeds 0.45 (twelve drinks if you only weigh 100 pounds), you stop breathing and DIE.

If you are routinely drinking enough to have memory gaps and/or pass out, *you have a problem.* This behavior is so risky both for your immediate health and the potential of what might happen to you while your judgment is so impaired—from drinking and driving to sexual assault. Imagine your younger sister/brother/niece/nephew choosing to drink till they pass out, and what could happen to them. In college health, we sadly see all the worst outcomes from the small subset of college students with a peer group where this is routine. Please talk with a counselor at your school if this seems to be the norm for you or your friend group.

Greeks, I'm especially talking to you—times are thankfully changing, and your national leadership is serious about revamping this dangerous culture. Truly, not "everyone" embraces alcohol abuse like this, and within every local Greek chapter, there should be student leaders willing to listen to your concerns, ready to help make practical changes within your chapter and pledge class. "Dry pledging" may be a fully acceptable and safer alternative, or it may simply lead you to other ridiculous or dangerous "tasks," depending on your frat. If you think something you are told to do is dangerous, risky, or just plain stupid, be the very empowered, ethical leader that your organization's mission touts and speak up—for you and your brothers/sisters.

Treatment:
Call 911 if the drunk person is:
- **Unconscious and vomiting**

- **Unconscious and breathing is irregular or slows to less than 8 breaths per minute**

  If someone is unconscious (passed out, you cannot wake them) but breathing regularly and not vomiting, use the Bacchus Maneuver to place them on their side and *stay with them.* If you have to leave or you might fall asleep, find someone else to be responsible, awake, and watching them.
- **Bacchus Maneuver:**

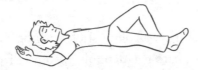

1. Position yourself on the person's right side and move their right arm up above their head.

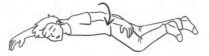

2. Reach across to their left shoulder and gently roll them toward you, being sure to protect their head from hitting the floor.

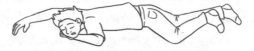

3. Tilt their head slightly up, using their left hand propped under their cheek (to keep their face off the floor). Stay with them till they are fully awake or medical professionals have arrived.

If someone is conscious and vomiting, stick around. Recognize their BAC may still be climbing, especially if they did shots.

Worst-case scenario:

Death. You already know that drunk driving kills too many people—twenty-nine people in the United States every day. But do you understand how being drunk can kill you directly?

If you're eating or drinking and accidentally swallow "wrong," what happens? Immediate, involuntary, and violent coughing until that tiny amount of liquid is out of your lungs. Alcohol poisoning suppresses your gag reflex, so if something goes "down the wrong pipe," instead of aggressively coughing, your body doesn't bother to respond . . . allowing you to choke on your own vomit, blocking your airway. Alternatively, high blood alcohol levels can slow and stop your drive to breathe, mess up your heart rhythm (including stopping the heart), or cause seizures.

Prevention:

- If you choose to drink alcohol, stick with beer or wine. While it is certainly possible to get alcohol poisoning from beer or wine, people rarely end up in the ER from those alone. Why?
  - **Volume**—most people feel uncomfortably full when they drink large amounts of beer and automatically slow down their consumption (versus the small physical volume of doing shots).
  - **Timely feedback**—rising blood alcohol levels cause progressive physical changes from the pleasant "buzz" and relaxation to impaired coordination to nausea, vomiting, and then passing out. Blood alcohol levels rise for about thirty to sixty minutes after you consume a drink. With beer and wine, most people drink slowly enough (one to two drinks per hour) that they feel the effects of rising blood alcohol levels in time to stop drinking and avoid the negative effects. Doing multiple shots in succession means your blood alcohol level hasn't had time to rise yet, so there's no early feedback to warn you.

TIPS:

- Ideally, limit yourself to one alcoholic drink per hour and decide your total limit *before* you start drinking.
- Drink something that you open yourself. A bottle or can of beer or a bottle of wine is ideal.

o Never drink on an empty stomach (because alcohol is absorbed more quickly, raising your blood alcohol levels faster).

o Don't drink while ADHD medications are in your system because you won't feel the normal signs of alcohol building up in your system.

  o See "ADHD Pre-Gaming" section in Chapter 8: Stimulants 101 (page 51).

o Drink a full glass of water (or other noncaffeinated, nonalcoholic drink like Sprite, sparkling water, juice, or Gatorade) after every alcoholic drink.

o **Drink Spiking:** If you have only had a couple drinks and suddenly you feel room-spinning nausea, vomiting, or intense intoxication, you have probably consumed a spiked drink. Tell a trusted friend **immediately** and ask them to take you to an ER, where you should request drug testing.

  o *The most common "spike" is more alcohol.* Adding clear, minimal-taste liquors to other drinks is still drink spiking if the recipient is unaware.

  o Additionally, prescription drugs like alprazolam (Xanax) or pain killers like hydrocodone (Vicodin) can easily be slipped into drinks. These drugs combined with alcohol are incredibly risky because together they really suppress your body's drive to breathe.

  o "Date-rape" drugs like GHB, Ketamine, and Rohypnol also find their way into seemingly benign drinks at parties. These drugs do not stay in your system very long, and the only way to find out is immediate drug testing, so do **not** wait till "tomorrow" morning.

    ➤ See Chapter 46: Date Rape & Sexual Assault (page 228).

Chapter 10

One Pill Can Kill: How to Recognize and Treat Opioid (Fentanyl) Overdose

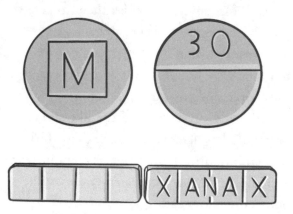

What If: You Find Someone Unconscious (Who May Have Unintentionally Taken Fentanyl)?

What most likely happened:

Scenario A: You're at a party where the music is pounding, virtually everyone's drinking, and some are obviously using other substances (weed, gummies, pills, etc.). You glance over to the side and notice someone rather awkwardly splayed across a couch, not moving much, appearing passed out. Although you're honestly not sure what to do, you decide to walk over and check on them, getting more anxious as you approach . . .

Scenario B: Your roommate has been super stressed out and not sleeping for at least a week. While getting ready for bed, they mention a friend gave them some "Xanax" so they can finally get some rest. You've been on your phone scrolling through social media for fifteen or twenty minutes when suddenly you are startled to hear your roommate snoring loudly, almost gasping, and when you get closer to check on them, you realize they are pale, clammy, unconscious, and struggling to breathe.

What's going on?

- In 2021, more than 80,000 Americans died from drug overdoses involving opioids, including more than 70,000 deaths from fentanyl, which is a pain medication that is 50 to 100 times stronger than morphine. *Over 90 percent of fentanyl deaths are thought to be ACCIDENTAL.* What does that mean? It means that the victim INTENTIONALLY took a pill they believed to be a known commodity, such as prescription alprazolam (Xanax), but that pill was actually an illegally manufactured drug tainted with a lethal dose of fentanyl. While virtually everyone is aware of the fentanyl crisis, it is easy to believe that this issue affects "them, not us" . . . until it tragically impacts your friends or your campus.
- Fentanyl (like other opioids such as morphine, oxycodone, and hydrocodone) creates a euphoric state of happiness and confidence while relieving pain, relaxing your body, and sedating your brain.
- Opioids can also cause nausea, vomiting, confusion, and a decreased drive to breathe.
- Signs of OPIOID OVERDOSE include:
  - Unresponsive/unconscious
  - Tiny, constricted pupils
  - Cold, clammy, pale skin
  - Blue lips or fingers
  - Nausea, vomiting

- Shallow, slow, or difficulty breathing (possibly gasping, snoring, or choking)
- Slow heart rate
- Limp body

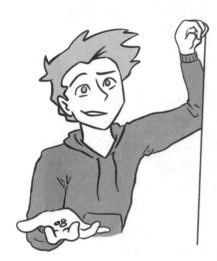

Here is what you REALLY need to know: College drug dealers *do not look scary*; they are usually your fellow students. That clean-cut, good-looking, friendly guy down the hall offering you an "Adderall" to keep you focused through your all-nighter for that term paper is a drug dealer. So is the girl in your class (or in your sorority, on your intramural team, or a fellow volunteer, etc.) who heard you fretting about not being able to sleep and offered you a "Xanax."

Even Drug Enforcement Agency experts cannot tell by looking whether a prescription medication is legitimate or fake, because drug cartels use imprinting machines to add the same alphanumeric markings on their pills as pharmaceutical companies. The most common fake prescription drugs are "Oxy" (Oxycontin), Xanax, Percocet, Vicodin, and Adderall.

Most student dealers would NEVER describe themselves as drug dealers! They typically slip into selling pills or weed simply to cover the cost of the substances they use themselves. Their conscience is eased by believing they are helping others focus, relax, or sleep. These young adults would never *intentionally* give someone a pill that might be lethal. Frankly, they are often in serious denial or have a somewhat understandable false sense of security about the risks because they are literally using the same drugs from the same source. Unfortunately, the fact is that the majority (up to 80 percent) of street drugs in the United States are now tainted with fentanyl. *Tragically, 6 out of 10 of these pills laced with fentanyl contain a potentially deadly dose.*

Why would drug dealers include enough fentanyl in their pills to kill their customers? Isn't that a terrible business plan?

- Fentanyl is added to street drugs because it takes a tiny amount to create the high, making it cheaper and easier to add or produce than any other opioids.
- Fentanyl is HIGHLY addictive, so lacing other drugs with minute amounts of fentanyl creates more addicts, therefore increasing the demand for their drugs.
- When you are addicted to an opioid drug, you become tolerant, meaning that it takes progressively more and more of the drug to achieve a similar high. A habitual user might be able to handle an amount of fentanyl that would kill a first-time user. Ironically, therefore, **overdose deaths can enhance the reputation of a dealer** because it implies their drugs are stronger than those of other dealers.
- Illegal fentanyl simply does not have consistent "quality control"—the amount and concentration of fentanyl can vary significantly with each batch.
- Sadly, especially with social media increasing access to consumers, the supply of future customers is virtually unlimited compared to the subset they kill.

Treatment:

Naloxone is the only medication that can directly reverse the effects of an opioid overdose. In September 2023, Narcan OTC became the first over-the-counter naloxone nasal spray available without a prescription.

Narcan OTC comes as a single dose nasal spray. Never "prime" the pump to see if the medication is spraying properly, because there is only one dose inside of it!

IF YOU FIND SOMEONE WHO IS UNCON-SCIOUS or who has other symptoms of an opioid overdose, never hesitate to try naloxone! First, quickly roll them on to their back if they are not positioned that way. Open the packaging, take out the spray, and hold it with your thumb on the bottom of the plunger and your pointer and middle fingers on either side of the nozzle. Tilt their head back and place the nozzle all the way inside one side of the nose and firmly press the plunger with your thumb. Call 911 immediately and stay with the victim until the emergency response personnel arrive. They may ask you to start CPR *(don't worry, "compressions only" are fine if you are not CPR trained or if you are simply not comfortable giving breaths)* as well as to give additional doses of naloxone every two to three minutes (if there is limited or no response to the first dose). If the victim does respond and start to breathe on their own, roll them on to their left side.

Head to the doctor if:
- You are using opioids and are having withdrawal symptoms like cravings and sweating, or if you are getting frustrated that you cannot seem to stop using them.
- **Anyone given Narcan needs to be taken to the Emergency Room for further evaluation,** even if they "wake up" and seem more alert.
- **ALWAYS CALL 911** if you administer naloxone (Narcan OTC ®).

Worst-case Scenario
- **Death**
- Remember, "One pill can kill."

Prevention
Only take prescription medications that you have personally been prescribed by a doctor AND you have purchased directly from a pharmacy. Expect that any other prescription medications you are offered could be laced with fentanyl, *even if you like or trust the person offering it to you.*

Be prepared! Purchase at least one naloxone nasal spray for your first aid kit and make sure it is easily accessible. Consider carrying it with you in your backpack or purse if you will be at a party or other situation where you are more likely to witness an accidental opioid overdose.

TIPS:

○ **How do you know if someone is UNCONSCIOUS versus drunk, high, or sleeping?** If you cannot wake the person by shouting their name and shaking their shoulders or rubbing their sternum (breast bone), they are UNCONSCIOUS, and you need to call 911 immediately.

○ **Narcan OTC (naloxone) will NOT HURT someone who is unconscious for another reason other than opioid overdose.** Please err on the side of USING this spray. If they did not overdose on opioids, you will do no harm. If they DID overdose on opioids, you may literally save their life!

○ **Stimulants (like cocaine and ADHD medications or other amphetamines) and hallucinogens (like cannabis and LSD) give you EXTRA LARGE pupils, while opioids (like morphine and fentanyl) cause TINY pupils.** *However, never depend on seeing tiny pupils to decide whether or not to give Narcan!* People very often have multiple substances in their system that have opposing effects on pupil size.

○ **Good Samaritan Laws** vary by state, but nearly all states have adopted these laws to protect bystanders from criminal prosecution if they call 911 for medical assistance for a victim who may be experiencing a drug or alcohol overdose. Most colleges in the United States are adopting similar medical amnesty policies to encourage students to reach out for help without fear of any university disciplinary actions.

Chapter 11
Seizures

What If: You have a Seizure?
Medical Name: Epileptic Seizure

What most likely happened:

Scenario A: The last thing you remember, you were doing vodka shots at a party. You came to and found yourself lying on the floor, with everyone leaning over you and looking freaked out. "We called EMS, they should be here soon! You had a seizure!"

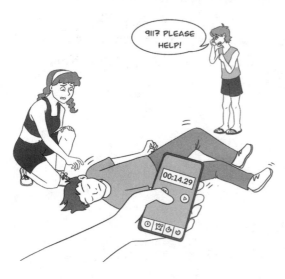

Scenario B: You've been super stressed out, not sleeping well, and thinking of changing majors because you hate organic chemistry and no longer want to go to medical school, plus you just ended your frustrating long-distance relationship with your high school sweetheart. Your doctor started you on a new antidepressant last week, and you feel twitchy and anxious, plus you can't shake the cough that's persisted after you had the flu, so you feel like you're living on cough syrup. As you were walking across campus to class, suddenly everything went black. As you woke up on the ground, you were vaguely aware you had lost control of your bladder and you were totally disoriented. Strangers are asking you questions and calling 911.

What's going on?

A seizure is a sudden, uncontrolled burst of electrical activity in the brain that can result in brief loss or alteration of consciousness, as well as convulsions. Note that one single seizure does not equal "epilepsy." The Epilepsy Foundation describes epilepsy as "a brain disorder that causes recurring, unprovoked seizures." In fact, we know that epilepsy is not a singular disorder but a diverse group of conditions that share a predisposition to recurrent, unprovoked seizures.

Epilepsy is far more common than you might expect; roughly 1 in 10 people in the United States will experience a seizure at some point during their lifetime, and 1 in 26 people will develop epilepsy (with "recurring, unprovoked seizures"). Roughly 1.2 percent of the United States' population has active epilepsy, which means they are either taking prescription seizure medication or have had at least one seizure in the past year.

COLLEGE STUDENTS have a HIGHER RISK of seizures than the general population, which is not surprising when you look at the triggers and risk factors.

Known triggers for seizures:
- **Alcohol:** acutely drinking too much (very common cause in college students) OR withdrawal after stopping heavy drinking
- **Street drugs**: especially amphetamines, cocaine, MDMA (ecstasy), and synthetic cannabinoids ("spice")
- **Prescription medications**: ADHD stimulant medications, antidepressants*, pain medications (tramadol), and isoniazid (an anti-tuberculosis medication)
- **Over-the-counter medications**: most commonly diphenhydramine (Benadryl)

- **Sleep deprivation** and **stress**
- **Flashing lights**
- **Head injury**
- **Very LOW or extremely HIGH blood sugar**—typically in diabetics
- **Very LOW (or less commonly, high) blood sodium levels, or low blood calcium or magnesium levels**
- **Infections** (especially meningitis, encephalitis, or a parasitic infection called cysticercosis)

*Note that ALL antidepressants can lower your seizure threshold (thus increasing your risk of having a seizure) and this is a major reason to strictly limit (or completely avoid) alcohol while taking antidepressants. Bupropion (brand name, Wellbutrin) carries the highest risk, at 0.4 percent incidence of seizures. The risk of having a seizure while on an antidepressant is directly related to the dose (risk increases as dose increases) as well as any other additional risk factors.

In COLLEGE STUDENTS, what we see most commonly are "PROVOKED SEIZURES." Otherwise healthy young adults with one or more baseline risk factors (such as sleep deprivation and/or being on an antidepressant) add in ANOTHER risk factor by binge drinking alcohol, using street drugs, or perhaps having allergy or cold symptoms that prompt them to take too much diphenhydramine (Benadryl) or cough syrup, and then the combination of all these risk factors ultimately push the brain beyond its threshold, provoking a seizure.

Treatment:
Provoked seizures MAY NOT require medications, but this is often a complex and challenging decision due to multiple risk factors that may have caused the seizure.

Medications: Prescription antiseizure medications are numerous; common ones include carbamazepine (Tegretol), phenytoin (Dilantin), oxcarbazepine (Trileptal), valproic acid (Depakote), topiramate (Topamax), gabapentin (Neurontin), lamotrigine (Lamictal), zonisamide (Zonegran), and levetiracetam (Keppra), among others.

AND . . . *something you may not have thought about . . .*

NO DRIVING! (for up to three to twelve months)
- **The driving restrictions are extremely complicated and vary significantly by state regulations, as well as by your doctor and the specifics of your circumstances.**
- Some states will not allow you to drive for a certain specified time after a seizure, regardless of the cause (including head injuries, infection, medications, alcohol, etc.).
- Additionally, in young adults, there are often multiple possible risk factors, which makes it difficult both medically and medicolegally for your physician to immediately "clear" you to drive, *even if they feel the seizure was provoked.*
- Some states have mandatory Department of Motor Vehicles physician reporting requirements for any patients with seizures; however, the vast majority of states expect people to voluntarily self-report.
- US state-mandated seizure driving restrictions are most commonly three to six months, but the range is "no set period" to eighteen months.

Initial Evaluation of a Seizure:
- First-time seizures need to be evaluated by a physician (most commonly in an Emergency Room) to look for brain injuries or underlying medical conditions that could be causing the seizure.
- A full neurological exam includes testing reflexes, muscle strength, coordination, cognition, memory, balance, and cranial nerve function. This exam will help the doctor determine if all the parts of your brain and the peripheral nerves in your body are functioning properly and can suggest whether or not there may be a structural problem in your nervous system.

- An EEG (Electro-Encephalo-Gram) is a test that measures the electrical activity of the brain. This is a painless study where electrodes are placed on the scalp to assess electrical impulses and look for bursts of activity that suggest seizures.
- An ECG (Electro-Cardio-Gram) is a heart tracing that checks for abnormal heart rhythms that could have made you faint/pass out.
- A CT scan is often used initially to look for tumors or any brain bleeding if there was any head trauma before the seizure.
- MRI scans help look for structural changes, brain tumors, or blood vessel malformations.
- Blood tests will look for anemia (low red blood cell count), low or high blood sugar levels, and any electrolyte abnormalities that may have triggered a seizure.
- Expect a urine and/or blood drug screen.

Head to your doctor (emergently) if:
- This is your first seizure.
- You have a known seizure disorder, but your seizure lasted longer than five minutes, or if witnesses say you had a second seizure after the first one ended.
- You were injured during your fall or the seizure itself (head, body, or extremities).
- You are diabetic.
- You are pregnant.
- You have any trouble breathing or can't seem to fully recover consciousness in five to ten minutes after your seizure ended.

Worst-case Scenario:
- If you fell and hit your head (before or even during the seizure), the worst-case scenario is a bleed inside your skull, on or in the brain.
- Brain tumors can show up as new onset seizures, but they are thankfully rare in young adults.

- Status epilepticus is a seizure that goes on too long—longer than five minutes, or when seizures occur so close together that the person does not awaken between seizures. This is a medical EMERGENCY that can lead to brain damage or, rarely, even death.
- SUDEP: Sudden Unexpected Death in EPilepsy occurs in people with epilepsy who are otherwise healthy. SUDEP is the most common cause of death in people with poorly controlled seizures. The best way to prevent SUDEP is to consistently take your medications and follow all the seizure control strategies recommended by your physician and health-care team.

Prevention:

- Always wear a helmet for protection to reduce head trauma during sports and recreational activities.
- Avoid mixing OTC cold medications with alcohol or antidepressant medications.
- NEVER use street drugs (remember, they are rarely "pure" and the contaminants typically lower your seizure threshold, among other concerns).
- Secondary prevention (after an initial seizure) includes adding in antiseizure medications. After your first adult seizure, you carry a significantly increased risk (between 21 to 45 percent) of having an additional seizure during the next two years. Note that if you are untreated (not given any antiseizure medication) and the seizure was UNPROVOKED, that risk increases even higher, to 40 to 50 percent. Obviously, this is why driving is restricted.

TIPS:

o In roughly 10 percent of the population, **FAINTING can lead to brief muscle twitching, which is technically a type of "provoked seizure" but is NOT considered EPILEPSY.** In medical terms, "vasovagal syncope" (fainting) can turn into a "convulsive syncope" when the temporarily decreased blood flow to the brain lowers oxygen levels enough to cause brief hypoxia that, in turn, provokes convulsive jerking movements. Thankfully, this fainting reaction quickly begins to reverse itself once the person is on the ground, because positionally, blood flow is faster to the brain in the prone position (versus standing and fighting gravity). We see convulsive syncope most often in our phlebotomy lab, where anxious students occasionally faint before or during blood draws. *If you tend to feel light-headed when you have your blood drawn, please let the staff know ahead of time.* Most clinics will have a spot where you can lie down rather than sit during your blood draw, which should help prevent any injury if you do faint.

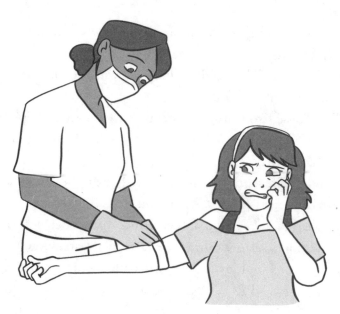

○ Be aware when traveling that **countries outside the United States have higher incidence of seizures**, largely from infectious sources such as bacterial meningitis, viral encephalitis, parasitic illnesses like cysticercosis, toxoplasmosis, and malaria.

○ People experiencing a seizure often **lose control of their bowel or bladder** (during the seizure, not a long-term issue but can be an immediate practical concern).

○ **NEVER try to put something in the mouth of a person experiencing a seizure!** This was an old intervention thought to keep people from biting or "swallowing" their tongue, but now we know that causes more harm than benefit.

If you see someone having a seizure, do these FOUR things. Remember, if you are not alone, ask other individuals to perform a specific task so everything happens ASAP.

1. **Top priority is to clear the space around the seizing person** (to avoid additional injuries) and, **if needed, ease them to the ground** if they have fallen on top of something like a chair/desk/bush/etc. If you have a jacket, pillow, or blanket handy, it's fine to try to slip that under their head to protect them from hitting their head on the ground.

2. **If possible, roll them onto their side** to limit choking or aspirating if they vomit.

3. *Unless you know the person has diagnosed epilepsy* (look for a medical warning bracelet), **CALL 911** and let them know you are witnessing a seizure.

4. **START COUNTING. Try the classic steady chant of "One, Mississippi, Two, Mississippi, Three . . ." or quickly activate the stopwatch on a phone or watch.** *When you are watching a seizure, it feels like it's going on FOREVER, but usually they last 30 to 120 seconds.* It's very helpful to medical providers to know exactly how long the seizure lasted.

Board Certified Neurologist Dr. Ayushi Chugh emphasizes, "TIME is BRAIN! If you think someone is having a seizure, protect them from injury, lay them on their left side, and call 911 immediately. *The longer the time a person is seizing, the greater the number of neurons (brain cells) that are lost,* leading to irreversible changes in their brain function, memory, and personality, which can lead to various psychosocial problems."

Chapter 12
Smoking, Vaping, and What You Might Not Know about Weed

What If: I Start Smoking, Vaping, or Using Weed?

Obviously, you know smoking is bad for you, and you likely grew up thinking cigarettes are disgusting . . . yet now you're vaping. Or maybe you've progressed beyond e-cigs to traditional cigarettes, which you know cause multiple cancers, heart attacks, and strokes. Pro tip: smoking anything (including vaping) also causes bad breath, stained teeth, and weakened, damaged tooth enamel that increases gum disease, tooth decay, and cavities. So, what made you start smoking? Odds are high the answer is an e-cig like JUUL or another vaping device. Nearly one-third (30.7 percent) of teens who use e-cigs will start smoking traditional cigarettes within six months.

Nicotine

No, nicotine alone doesn't cause cancer, but *nicotine doesn't travel alone.* Traditional cigarettes contain over sixty known carcinogens, and e-cigs combine nicotine with metals like nickel, cadmium, and chromium plus volatile organic compounds and flavorings that directly cause acute and chronic lung inflammatory disease. No question that vaping is bad for your lungs, though we will need at least another decade to start assessing the full cancer risks.

Vaping (or smoking) rapidly shoots nicotine into the bloodstream, where it races to the adrenal glands and releases adrenaline, which causes the physical "rush" of racing heart, elevated blood pressure, and faster breathing. Your brain interprets this body response as excitement and joy, while at the cellular level, the nicotine triggers the pleasure/reward circuits via dopamine stimulation. This response all happens within ten seconds after inhalation, creating a brief euphoria that rapidly disappears, leaving the body craving more . . . and the cycle begins.

Students often begin using vaping devices like JUUL as an easily accessible caffeine substitute, taking a hit before a test or a steady drip of hits to stay focused while studying. Others use it to suppress appetite or catch a "confidence buzz" without calories.

- Does it work? In the short term, yes. That's what hooks you.
- Is it worth it? **No.**

Nicotine (like caffeine) can suppress your appetite, give you a few minutes of "feel good," and transiently improve concentration and memory. However, repeated exposure to nicotine quickly goes beyond the short-term buzz to adversely affect higher-level brain circuits like learning processes and impulse control. Continued usage also requires more nicotine to get that same pleasure and bodily response, and soon merely the *lack of nicotine creates withdrawal symptoms* of cravings, agitation, sleep disturbance, poor concentration, and irritability. This is **nicotine physical dependence**, which happens quickly for most people; and although there are clearly individual sensitivities (and those lucky few who can easily quit), this is not a substance to casually "try." The majority of adult smokers want to quit, and half actively try to quit each year (though many are not successful). The more you use nicotine, the less it works; the more you need, the more you use . . . and **nicotine addiction** (compulsively using nicotine despite knowing it is harming you) is the result. A meta-analysis showed 40 percent can quit cocaine, 18 percent can quit alcohol, but only 8 percent can quit smoking.

- E-cigs randomly explode, and in the FEMA U.S. Fire Administration report, 30 percent of the explosions occurred while the device was being used and another 30 percent occurred while the device was in a pocket. These explosions not surprisingly resulted in extensive burn injuries. The remaining explosions were reported while the device was charging (24%), being stored (9%), or transported (<1%).
- Some people vape to "sober up" after drinking. News flash: Stimulants like caffeine and nicotine don't "undo" sedatives like alcohol or pot, *they simply make you a more awake and agitated intoxicated person*. Your reflexes and reaction times are still impaired. Please do NOT drive.
- Nicotine addiction is **expensive**: $5–20/disposable vape or pod or $9/pack of cigs will quickly deplete your bank account.

Cannabis

Recreational cannabis products are legal in many states, and frankly, they are readily available for those seeking them in every state, on virtually every campus. An estimated 8 percent of college students use cannabis daily, and 43.6 percent of college students admit to using cannabis at least once within the last year *(which means 92 percent do NOT use daily and over half of college students have not used any in the last year)*. Interestingly, studies consistently show that college students believe a much higher percent of their peers are using cannabis products than are actually doing so, which certainly could be a skewed perception due to friend group usage. The fact is that **not "everyone" is using weed**. Also, consider the following:

- **If you didn't grow it, you don't know what's in it** (*especially if you are purchasing outside of a legal dispensary*). Frequently, when people have a "bad trip" with consequences that send them to the ER or our urgent care, they believe they "only" used weed yet their drug screens show not only cannabis, but unexpected other drugs (like LSD). Illegal drug dealers continually search for ways to cheaply make their weed stronger, more hallucinogenic—and they don't mind adding in a pinch of formaldehyde, acid, or other dangerous chemicals to do so. Additionally, since weed is sold by the gram/ounce, some add sand and glass particles to increase the weight, which increases irritation and damage to your lungs. We've seen harmful contaminants in the vaping fluid. In 2019, there was a thankfully short-lived epidemic of "e-cigarette or vaping product use-associated lung injury" (EVALI) that resulted in sixty-eight deaths and over 2800 hospitalizations of otherwise healthy young people. The culprit turned out to be innocent-sounding Vitamin E acetate, which was used as a dilutional agent. *Buyer beware!*

- **Regular cannabis use impairs short-term memory, judgment, motivation, and learning** . . . not brilliant for college success. Additionally, THC can slow down your brain's ability to learn, process, and store new information in your long-term memory for up to twenty-four hours; so last night's edibles are not helping this morning's study session. Studies show frequent cannabis users have lower GPAs, skip class more, and take longer to graduate.

- **This is not "your parent's pot"!** THC (tetrahydro cannabidiol) is what makes you "high." In the 1970s, the THC concentration in cannabis averaged 2 to 4 percent. Today's "weed" has an average THC concentration of 15 percent, and cannabis extracts used in edibles, dab, oil, and "shatter" can range from 50 to above 90 percent. *These high-potency products come with a whole new level of risk for addiction, mood disorders, and psychosis.*

- Today's cannabis has clear and often intense symptoms of withdrawal, including powerful cravings for more cannabis, anxiety, insomnia, irritability, and feelings of unease and dissatisfaction, *which mimic many of the reasons many use cannabis in the first place.* Ultimately, this creates a vicious cycle of use, transient relief, withdrawal symptoms, craving, using more THC to seek relief . . . and repeat. Students very often start using weed at night to "calm their brain" and help them fall asleep, but before long they are addicted, and then their withdrawal symptoms actually make their insomnia worse.

- **What about "casual" use? One in six teens (17 percent) and one in eleven adults (9 percent) won't be able to keep it "casual," because they will become dependent on cannabis.** Brains younger than age twenty-five are massively remodeling, which makes them more susceptible to addiction. Adolescent brains intensively improve and reshape, adding white matter to speed communication and "pruning" away less effective connections until roughly age twenty-five. The final area to develop is our prefrontal cortex—the site of executive functions like decision making, impulse control, understanding consequences, and problem solving. Cannabis use (as well as heavy alcohol use or prolonged daily video gaming) disrupts and impairs this process, preventing your brain from reaching its maximum potential.
- **Federal law states: "recreational and medical use of cannabis is illegal."**
    - Although many states have legalized cannabis, FEDERAL LAW still prohibits the manufacture, distribution, dispensation, and possession of cannabis other than in approved research studies.
    - Even in states that have legalized cannabis, it is STILL ILLEGAL for anyone UNDER THE AGE OF TWENTY-ONE to *buy, have or use cannabis.*
    - Note that it is a FELONY to GIVE, SHARE, or SELL cannabis to anyone under the age of twenty-one.

You have likely heard of getting the "munchies" from cannabis, but are you aware of Cannabinoid Hyperemesis Syndrome (CHS)? This relatively uncommon but serious problem typically develops in otherwise healthy, long-term, daily cannabis users. CHS may start with days or weeks of frequent "morning sickness" or vague stomach discomfort and can suddenly evolve into a relentless cycle of intense nausea and persistent vomiting so severe that treatment requires hospitalization.

Anne F. Liu, MD, Lecturer in Harvard Medical School's Division of Gastroenterology, Hepatology, and Endoscopy, has seen a significant increase in this problem, and asks these three questions to help her identify patients:

- Do you shower or bathe multiple times in one day?
- When you do shower, do you crank the heat up as high as possible?
- How long do you stay in the shower?

If the answers are yes, yes, and basically "until the hot water runs out," Cannabinoid Hyperemesis Syndrome is almost certainly the cause.

Dr. Liu explains that cannabis slows down the speed with which food exits the stomach and moves into the intestine, while at the same time triggering receptors in the brain that make us puke. Additionally, THC can fool the brain into thinking the body is cold, which prompts patients to seek a warmer skin temperature. This is why we see severe vomiting and compulsive desire for hot water on the skin in CHS.

Cannabinoid Hyperemesis Syndrome is challenging to diagnose. Both patients and clinicians often initially think food poisoning or a bad "stomach flu" is to blame, and patients may be treated and sent home, only to return to the ER with persistent symptoms. Blood tests show no signs of infection, nor do they reveal any consistent abnormalities with the liver, pancreas, thyroid, kidneys, etc. that might more commonly explain the nausea. If the patient has an endoscopy to look for obstructions or other issues in the GI tract, this is typically normal as well. *The only way to diagnosis and treat CHS is to discover that the patient has been chronically using cannabis (which many people are hesitant to discuss), and the only cure is for the patient to permanently stop using it—with the help of short-term hospitalization, IV fluids, and anti-nausea medications.*

What about EDIBLES?

- These innocent-appearing gummies, brownies, or chocolate often appeal to people who have never tried weed, partly because there is no need to smoke or inhale anything, and partly because these mimic familiar products. Truly, who's afraid of a gummy bear or candy bar?
- **Before you take that first bite:**
    - You will NOT feel the buzz for a minimum of thirty minutes, and likely not for an hour or more!
    - Too much THC can cause nausea, vomiting, panic, anxiety, or psychosis (like paranoia).
    - The recommended recreational "serving" is 2.5mg for first-time users (max 5 mg), which is a FRACTION of the edible—like 1 square of a chocolate bar or ¼ or ½ of a single GUMMY!
    - **The most common mistake** is to eat "just one more" gummy or "just another bite or two" of the cookie, because you aren't feeling anything after ten, twenty, or thirty minutes—which then results in over-intoxication an hour later.
    - Mixing alcohol or stimulants with edibles is risky and very likely to worsen the adverse effects of over-consumption— don't do it.

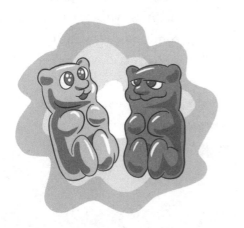

    - Do NOT plan on driving home— significant THC effects last for up to twelve hours.
    - **"Weed (and/or gummies) helps my anxiety."** In an isolated situation, this may be true (although note it can also exacerbate anxiety, add irritability and/or paranoia, or cause a panic attack). Regularly escaping anxiety with mind-altering substances

rather than learning healthy coping skills (talking with others, exercise, meditation, music, art) stunts your psychological maturation in addition to the THC messing with your prefrontal cortex and final brain development. Ultimately, studies and clinical experience show that using weed (or alcohol) to calm your nerves is at best a temporary solution that ultimately yields worse outcomes for anxiety and depression.

- **Internships & Jobs.** Major companies often drug test their employees, *including summer interns.* How long does THC stay in your system? Depends how much you consume, how often, and your weight—specifically your fat concentration, because THC is stored in fat. A nonsmoker who smokes weed one time may have a positive urine test for a few days; a "casual" weekend user tests positive for about a week; a daily cannabis user may test positive on a urine test for over a month. *Hair sample testing, however, may remain positive for up to three months.* Nothing ruins graduation weekend like flunking a drug test and losing that dream job you worked so hard to achieve.

  - **Quitting** may be much harder than you expect, especially if you've become a daily user. Seek help from your counseling center early—please don't wait till April of your senior year!
  - **Never count on a urine drug screen**. All those products you see advertised to "clean" your urine may sometimes help cheat a urine test, but nothing will "clean" your hair.

Chapter 13
Freshman Fifteen
(An Ounce of Prevention)

What If: I'm Worried about Gaining the Freshman Fifteen?

Weight gain in college is obviously restricted neither to freshmen nor to "fifteen" pounds, but gaining weight is a common problem, and the first semester is typically the worst time.

Why do students gain weight?

- Stopping or dramatically dropping intensity level of your often lifelong sport/dance/martial arts/marching band
- First time you are completely and solely responsible for what, when, and where you eat, so nearly half of freshmen change their established eating habits
- Socializing focuses around high-calorie convenience and delivery foods (pizza, burgers, shakes, sodas, chips, cookies)
- **Liquid calories**—sodas and alcohol add up quickly. Do the math:
  - 3,500 calories = 1 pound
  - Average **beer**: 150 kcal; **23 beers** = 1 pound of weight gain
  - Average **Vodka** shot: 90 kcal; **39 shots** = 1 pound

- **Margaritas:** 450–680 kcal; **6 average margaritas** = 1 pound
- **Soda:** 150 kcal; 23 sodas = 1 pound
- **Starbucks Frappuccino:** 190–530kcal
  - Grande (16 ounces): 300kcal; **12 frappes** = 1 pound
- Stress eating and drinking
- Study calories (Starbucks, energy drinks, and "reward" candy bars)
- "All you can eat"–style dining plans

Prevention:

- **Be aware**: Recognize routine extra calories "in" (new Starbucks habit) or fewer calories "out" (no longer in team practices) and make adjustments to balance your changing habits.
- Consider a **personal trainer** for twice-a-month sessions your first semester.
  - Most universities have very affordable, discounted personal training at their gyms.
- Join an **intramural sport** that fits your competitive level.
- **Accountability**: Either step on a scale or try on "those" nonstretch jeans once a week. If you (like many students) live in comfy large T-shirts and elastic-waist shorts or leggings, you may not realize you are steadily gaining weight.
- Use your phone, Fitbit, Apple watch, or similar product to keep track of your activity and calories burned.
- Find a fun exercise class (martial arts, Zumba, cross-training); ideally, grab a friend and commit to going together once or twice per week.
- Count your fruit and veggie servings; goal should be five to ten servings per day.
  - A serving is the size of your cupped hand
  - A salad might be four to six servings—this is very doable!
- Walk and talk with a friend (or listen to music) for study breaks rather than sitting and scrolling social media or playing games.

- Get enough **sleep**—at least seven to nine hours.
    - Studies prove that poor or reduced sleep can lead to weight gain!

TIPS:

○ **Liquid calories are the biggest culprit.** *If you make no changes in your exercise routine* and the only change in your diet is adding in one Starbucks per day, plus an average of six (alcoholic) drinks over each weekend . . . ***you will gain at least three pounds per month.***

○ If you choose more calories in, you need more calories out. (Duh!) But the tip is to **learn what you burn**—how many **actual** calories are going "out." Most people overestimate the calories they burn, thinking jogging two miles "buys" them a margarita, when it's only buying you half of that drink. Buyer beware!

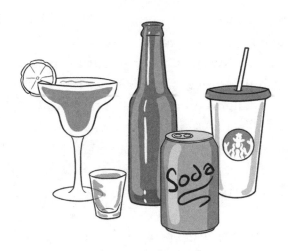

Chapter 14

Something's Stuck in My Eye

What If: Something's Stuck in My Eye?

Medical Name: Foreign Body & Possible Corneal Abrasion

What most likely happened:

Scenario A: After a late night of studying (or partying too much), you fell asleep (or passed out) without taking out your contacts. Waking up the next morning, your pry your aching eyes open, and now you can't even remove one of your contacts. The more you try to get it out, the worse it hurts and makes your eye spasm shut.

  Scenario B: Something scraped or flew into your eye—a tree branch, glitter, dust, a flake of mascara, or perhaps a finger. Or you rubbed your eyes really, really hard. You tried flushing it out and can't see anything still in there, but now your eye hurts intensely, tears are flowing, bright light makes it worse, and you can barely force your eye open.

What's going on?

You've irritated or scratched your cornea, the clear dome of tissue that covers your iris (the colored part of the eye, including over the pupil). Any corneal scratch is potentially serious, because the top layer of the cornea is so thin—only five to seven cell layers deep. Know that a dried-out contact can be literally stuck to your cornea, so pulling out the contact can rip the cornea. Don't force it!

Self-treatment:
- Try to flush out your eye with generous amounts of sterile saline (contact lens solution).
  - Avoid using bottled or tap water because those sources may contain microscopic organisms that can infect your eye.
  - If you have a stuck and dried-out contact lens, it may take up to fifteen minutes of repeated flushing to rehydrate that lens enough to release it from your cornea.
- Next, try pulling your top eyelid directly over the bottom lid and blink, thus using your own eyelashes as a brush to sweep underneath the top lid.
- Grab sunglasses to minimize further irritation from light and then get to a clinic.
  - Do **not** drive yourself (even if it's only one eye affected).
- Do **not** rub your eye or use any object like a Q-tip to try and remove debris.
- Do **not** use the "get the red out" eye drops.

Professional treatment:
- After assessing your vision (starting with the "Big E" chart), the first intervention is usually a numbing eye drop that will temporarily ease your pain, so your clinician can thoroughly examine your eye front to back, including under your eyelids, and try to remove any remaining debris.
  - Finding and removing glitter or other small objects may be simple and quick but is often challenging (particularly if you are having intense eye spasms).
- Next, a fluorescein stain is applied that sticks to and lights up any scratches on your cornea, revealing the exact size and position of your injury.

- If you have significant visual loss or a large corneal scrape, your care should continue with an ophthalmologist. Smaller injuries with minimal visual change may be managed by your primary care provider, but you should expect daily follow-up visits until your eye is healed.
- Eye patches are not typically recommended for this type of injury.
- Prescription medications:
    - Antibiotic eyedrops or eye ointment to prevent infection
    - Anti-inflammatory eyedrops to ease discomfort
- Although most small abrasions will heal in twenty-four to forty-eight hours, do not wear contacts again until your clinician clears you (typically at least a week) and definitely dispose of the ones you were wearing and start with a fresh set.

Head to your doctor if:
This one is simple—if you have a painful eye or blurred vision, especially if you wear contacts, go get checked out.

Worst-case scenario:

Blindness. Not to be overly dramatic, but understand that this thin layer must remain clear, because this is literally your window to the world. Infections, inflammation, and erosion can cause discoloration and scarring, which may blur and possibly completely obscure your previously clear window. Therefore, any incomplete healing can leave you with blurred vision. The only cure for permanently damaged corneas is corneal transplant surgery.

Prevention:

- Say **no** to glitter! (*So not worth the Instagram pic of tossed glitter on Bid Day!*)
- Wear sunglasses outside, especially if you are biking or riding a scooter.
- Always wear protective goggles if working with chemicals, wood, or metal.

- **Do Not Ever** sleep with your contacts in. Yes, there are extended-wear lenses that advertise it's fine for you to sleep with them in, but just like dentists recommend and truly do floss every day, eye doctors recommend never sleeping with contacts in your eyes.
- If you don't have daily disposable lenses, set reminders on your phone to replace your extended wear disposable lenses as directed (usually every two weeks), and if your eyes are bothering you with scratchiness or discomfort, change them earlier and consider giving your eyes a break by wearing glasses for an afternoon.

TIPS:

○ **Bring your prescription glasses with you to college** even if you "never" wear them (because obviously if you scrape your eye, you have no other options).

○ **Painful** eyes need to be examined as soon as possible; do **not** try to tough it out.

○ The worst thing ophthalmologists see is people damaging their own eye trying to get a contact out *that actually fell out hours earlier.* The pain and "foreign body" sensation persists even when whatever was in there scraping your eye is gone. Don't go on a "fishing" expedition when you can't see anything!

○ Putting your contact in your mouth to "re-wet" it when you don't have lens solution with you is a **bad idea**; our mouths are full of germs you don't want to introduce to your eye (with possibly the worst being herpes simplex virus—HSV—that causes fever blisters/cold sores). Better to toss out the lens and start over if you get stuck in this situation.

○ If you wake up with normal vision but a scary-looking, **painless** bright red splotch on the white part of one eye after a night of strenuous coughing, sneezing, or prolonged vomiting, you likely ruptured a capillary blood vessel. Despite their dramatic appearance, these subconjunctival hemorrhages are usually medically insignificant.

Chapter 15
Zoom Fatigue

What If: You Suffer from "Zoom Fatigue"?
Medical name: Asthenopia (eye strain) plus cognitive and physical fatigue

What most likely happened:
You feel like you are more mentally drained and/or physically fatigued after online lectures in the comfort of your own room (and possibly pajamas) than when you had to get up, get dressed, and attend class in person. *Shouldn't it be less effort and therefore less tiring?* Nope!

What's going on?
"Zoom fatigue" (a.k.a. virtual fatigue) is far more than simple eye strain from looking at electronic screens. Your brain is juggling information non-stop, focusing attention on the speaker yet also darting around to inspect a variety of distractions. Meanwhile, your eyes are literally drying out from reduced blinking, while your neck, back, and shoulders have morphed into a C-shaped cluster of tense muscles. The good news is that once you understand why virtual learning is so exhausting, you can do many things to make it better.

Let's breakdown Zoom fatigue into each contributing factor, offering prevention tips and solution strategies with each issue:

Problem #1: Constant focus

As opposed to in-person classes or meetings, your attention (*or at least the appearance of your attention*) is *nonstop*. The next time you have an in-person conversation, notice how often you or your friend naturally shift your gaze or move your head and body as you chat. It's normal to frequently turn your head, glance, or react to your surroundings while still being fully engaged in your conversation. Contrast this with being an attentive online listener, where it's polite to maintain eye contact with the speaker (assuming you are on camera) and where

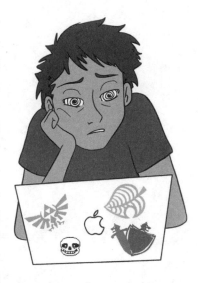

you often remain hunched in the same position in front of your laptop for the duration of the lecture. This degree of direct, focused attention is far more draining than "in real life."

Solutions:

- Mindfully shift your gaze and change your head position often.
- Change your position from leaning back in your chair with crossed arms to leaning forward with your chin propped on one or both hands, and/or include subtle changes like tilting your head to alternating sides.
- While you don't want to move so often that you appear squirmy or constantly fidgeting, a good rule of thumb is to be sure you aren't staying in the same exact position for more than roughly five minutes. Set your watch or phone to vibrate if you need a subtle reminder.

Problem #2: Self-attraction

Scientific studies prove that we are unconsciously drawn to looking at our own face. If your gorgeous face is visible in that upper right-hand corner, your brain literally keeps trying to focus on it and pull your attention away from the speaker.

Solution:

- Easy fix for this one on Zoom: Simply right-click on the box with the three dots in the top right corner of the video and choose "Hide self." *Poof!* Your face disappears.

Problem #3: Curiosity

Not only are we attracted to ourselves, but our attention is subconsciously diverted to examine other people's faces or perhaps to decipher background objects behind those faces.

Solutions:

- Start with maximizing the speaker and minimizing everyone else in the meeting.
- Try to be aware and refocus if you slip down the rabbit hole of reading book titles or scrutinizing pictures behind the speaker.
- If you are in a large enough class that it would not be rude, consider taking a timed two-minute visual break every fifteen to twenty minutes by either turning off your camera or simply closing your eyes (but continuing to listen).

Problem #4: Distractions

Deep down, *most of us honestly think that we are fully capable of multitasking while still listening and fully absorbing lecture content*, but this is a huge part of Zoom fatigue! If you are checking and responding to texts and emails or browsing social media, your brain is working hard to zip back and forth, constantly playing catch up on what it missed from either the speaker or that last work email. Let me be clear: if you are multitasking, *you are absolutely not learning and retaining information anywhere near full capacity.* Distracted learning is both inefficient and mentally exhausting.

Solutions:

- **Eliminate distractions before class begins!**
- Close out open tabs on your screen besides Zoom and necessary class links so you can fully commit your attention to class.
- Physically put your Switch or other gaming systems out of sight/ reach.
- Purposefully schedule ten-minute social media time into your day (right before or immediately after class works for many students) to help break the habit of checking Snapchat/Instagram/ Facebook/etc. during lectures.
- Consider deleting games from your phone (move them to your iPad or another computer tablet if that's an option) and only use your phone to text a classmate a comment or question as you would in person. Better yet, if you have a chat feature for class and you can put your phone out of reach and out of sight, do it.

Problem #5: Dry eyes

We blink far less than normal when fixating on screens (and especially if you are looking at multiple screens), so our eyes literally get dried out, causing discomfort that ranges from dull aching to burning, stinging, or light sensitivity and possibly blurred vision. Ironically, dry eyes can also cause excessive tearing as part of your body's response to that dryness.

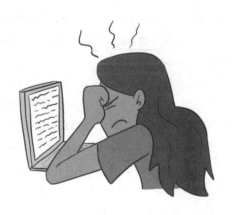

Solutions:

- Try to alternate using glasses instead of contacts if you need prescription vision correction.
- Whether or not you need glasses/contacts, try applying rehydrating eye drops between classes (NOT "get the red out"

ones, but moisturizing artificial tear–style products within brands like Refresh, Systane, Blink, or Thera Tears). Remember to sanitize and air-dry your hands before using!

- For extra dry eyes, consider a five-minute eye break by using a product like Refresh Celluvisc gel. Note that products like this will blur your vision for a few minutes, so don't apply at the start of a class.
  - *If you wear contacts, talk with your doctor about specific products and timing of application, because you can only use basic rewetting/moisturizing drops when your contacts are in place.*

Problem #6: "Turtle" neck

As the hours drag on sitting in front of your laptop, you may find your head sinking down and your shoulders migrating upward toward your ears until you end up with a highly un-ergonomic, super-scrunched, and uncomfortably distorted head, neck, and upper-body posture. Laptop computers create an unnatural forced neck flexion that can increase the effective weight of your head from nearly ten pounds at a neutral position to a shocking sixty pounds at sixty degrees of flexion. This constant flexion weakens your neck and back (especially trapezius and rhomboid) muscles, worsening your head-forward posture, which further strains your muscles and creates a negative loop. Treatment starts with stretching and strengthening exercises, but that will only be a band-aid if you don't fix the basic problem, which is the ergonomic dysfunction from the abnormal laptop posture.

Solutions:

- **MOVE between classes**. Every single, solitary break, make yourself get up out of your chair, couch, or bed and walk around, do something like jumping jacks or dance moves, grab some water or a snack, and stretch, stretch, stretch!
- If you have extended or back-to-back classes, set your watch or phone timer to vibrate every twenty minutes to remind you to shift positions, stand, or subtly stretch.

TIPS:

- ○ **Dress for success.** Consider getting ready for an online class as you would for one in person, meaning literally shower and get dressed, and sit at a table or your desk, rather than lounging on your bed. Radio broadcasters have taught this prep technique for years in media training for recording their call-in, out-of-studio radio show guests. *Even when you know you won't be seen, "presenting" yourself as though you were in-person makes you far more mentally alert.*

- ○ Zoom fatigue is ultimately the result of *lack of physical movement* combined with excessive *mental gymnastics.* The more you can encourage your body to naturally move (from blinking, to shifting your head and body) and the less jumping around your brain needs to do to focus on the speaker, the better you will learn and perform.

Chapter 16
Stye, Stye, in My Eye

What If: I Have a Stye?
Medical name: Hordeolum

What most likely happened:
Inevitably, the day before your big date/interview/photo shoot, you wake up to find a tender red bump or what looks like a pimple (red bump with a white head on it) right on the edge or just below your eyelid along the eyelashes. Often the lid will swell up as well, and sometimes it can be difficult to see the actual stye on your own. Your vision should not be affected (unless your lid is so swollen that it is blocking the pupil), and typically this only affects one eye at a time.

What's going on?
Bacteria or debris (especially from mascara or other eye makeup) can enter the eyelash follicles and ultimately block the oil glands, causing the swelling and pimple appearance. Styes may be internal or external. To see an internal stye, you may need to gently pull down or evert/flip out the lid, whereas external styes are easily seen along the base of your eyelashes.

Treatment:
The vast majority of styes will resolve on their own, within a week to ten days, often more quickly if moist heat is religiously applied. Classic

treatment is moist heat with a washcloth soaked in warm water (not so hot it burns you, of course) held firmly on your eye for multiple ten-minute sessions, rewetting it as soon as you no longer feel the moist heat. Repeat this process several times per day, basically as often as you can. Antibiotics (both oral and topical preparations like drops or ointments) do not speed up healing of common styes, nor do over-the-counter eyedrops or ointments.

When to head to your doctor:
- Any change in your vision
- Eyelid completely swollen shut
- Any blisters on the eyelid (this could be shingles or another herpes infection)
- If your symptoms are not improving after a few days (or if swelling increases)

Worst-case scenario:

Occasionally, persistent styes require minor surgical intervention from an ophthalmologist to speed up healing, and at that point, topical antibiotics may be added, but this is the exception, definitely not the rule.

Simple styes can progress to become a more complicated medical condition called a chalazion, which looks like a flesh-colored bigger bump more toward the center of the eyelid, usually the upper lid. Chalazion treatment may take weeks to months and includes topical and/or oral antibiotics, steroid injections, and, if necessary, ultimately surgical intervention from an ophthalmologist.

Prevention:

Eyelid scrubs are a great way to maintain good eye hygiene, especially for those who wear eye makeup that includes mascara. Either buy commercial disposable individual eyelid wipes or keep a small bottle of baby shampoo on your sink (or take it to your shower) and use a small drop on your fingertips to gently massage the base of your eyelashes after you have washed your face and removed makeup; massage for about ten seconds, then rinse with copious amounts of water.

Replace your mascara every few months and start with a new tube to minimize bacterial contamination, and **never** share mascara with others. (Consider sharing mascara like sharing a toothbrush: Just. Say. **No.**) NEVER put eyeliner on your "waterline"! The area below your upper lashes and above your lower lashes is not "skin," it's a membrane that houses tiny oil glands. These Meibomian oil glands secrete oil and create a tear film to keep our eyes moist, and when you block them, not only will you get a stye, but you may also end up with dry eyes and blurry vision.

TIPS:

○ "It's not the **Degree**, it's the **Duration** that matters!"
  ○ Do not try to make the heat as high as you can stand it, but instead focus on doing the warm compresses for the full ten or even fifteen minutes and repeat them three or four times per day.
  ○ Consider making a **"rice sock"** homemade moist heat heating pad by putting a cup of uncooked rice (not the instant-minute variety, but uncooked grains) into a cotton sock, tie a knot in the sock to keep the rice inside, then heat in the microwave for thirty to sixty seconds. The heated rice sock will hold moist heat longer than a warm washcloth. **Caution:** *Microwaves heat unevenly, so carefully check that the sock is not too hot before holding it up to your face.*
○ **Resist the temptation** to squeeze or "pop" the stye. Trust me, this only leads to more swelling and complications and does **not** help your stye disappear faster.

Chapter 17
Pink Eye: Infectious or Allergic?

What If: I Get "Pink Eye"?
Medical Name: Conjunctivitis

What most likely happened:
Scenario A: You woke up with one eye matted shut *(or occasionally both eyes, though usually one is worse than the other)*, and after wiping off the dried gunk, now your eyes are red, irritated, or stinging, and one eye seems to be churning out more of the watery or mucus-appearing discharge. Your vision may be temporarily blurry, but it clears with blinking, and light should not hurt your eyes. Your eyes may feel gritty, but they are not intensely painful.

    Scenario B: A runny nose and sneezing have plagued you all week, and now both eyes have become extremely itchy, with stringy "sleep" (discharge) in your eyes, and your eyelids may be a bit swollen. Once again, vision is unchanged and this is uncomfortable, but no sharp pain.

What's going on?
In both scenarios, tiny blood vessels are inflamed in the clear outer layer that covers the white part of your eyes. That layer is called the conjunctiva,

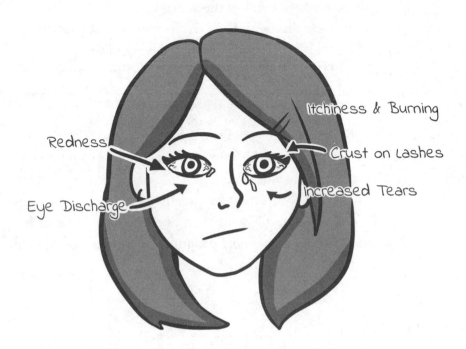

Redness

Eye Discharge

Itchiness & Burning

Crust on Lashes

Increased Tears

and "-itis" means inflammation, so this is conjunctivitis. Scenario A describes an infection, whereas B is an allergic response. Both cases cause red or "pink" discoloration in the white part of your eyes.

Viral conjunctivitis is the most frequent culprit in adults, and often mixed in with common cold symptoms like nasal congestion and sore throat. This is the classic "pink eye" everyone fears because of the highly contagious nature of this infection, and outbreaks often occur in the community, especially during the summer.

- The typical eye discharge is watery, and you may feel a swollen lymph node (feels like a firm pea) directly in front of your ear or under your chin.
- Symptoms often start in one eye then show up in the other eye a day or two later.
- Common cold symptoms like nasal congestion or sore throat may start before, during, or after the eye symptoms.

- Lids are often very swollen, but the actual discharge volume is typically much less than with bacterial infections. Additionally, when the lids are gently "pried" open by the examining physician, the "whites" of the eye will appear less inflamed and red compared with bacterial conjunctivitis.

Bacterial conjunctivitis tends to cause enough discharge to stick the eyelids together in the morning, and this infection is both more common and more serious in contact lens wearers.

Allergic conjunctivitis occurs most frequently in the spring and summer, triggered by tiny airborne allergens such as tree pollens, animal fur, mold, or dust mites. Itching is the most prominent symptom, along with small amounts of stringy white discharge.

Treatment:
- **Viral pink eye:**
  - Symptomatic relief only
  - Use artificial tears
  - Apply moist, warm compresses to remove dried eye discharge
  - Ophthalmologist Julia Sargent, MD, strongly advises, "**Stay home!** You are highly contagious so please don't head to class and expose everyone around you."
- **Bacterial pink eye:**
  - Topical antibiotics are prescribed if symptoms persist more than one day or if initial symptoms are severe.
  - Use warm compresses as needed to remove dried discharge.
- **Allergic pink eye:**
  - Many different types of prescription eyedrops are available that may be more effective with fewer side effects than oral medications. Common choices include:
    - Antihistamine drops:
      - Azelastine (Optivar)
    - Mast Cell Stabilizer drops:

- Nedocromil (Alocril)
- Pemirolast (Alamast)
- Lodoxamine (Alomide)
- Cromolyn (Crolom)
- Combo antihistamine/mast cell stabilizer drops:
  - Olopatadine (Patanol/Pataday)
  - Epinastine (Elestat)
  - Ketotifen (Zaditor/ Alaway)
  - NonSteroid Anti-Inflammatory Drug (NSAID)
  - Ketorolac (Acular)
- Steroid drops:
  - Loteprednol (Lotemax, Alrex)
- Oral antihistamines like loratadine (Claritin), fexofenadine (Allegra), or cetirizine (Zyrtec) may also provide relief.
- Seasonal allergy nasal steroid sprays like triamcinolone acetonide (Nasacort) or fluticasone (Flonase) may also offer improvement in eye symptoms.
- Looking for a compress? Use **cold compresses**, not hot.

Is it viral or bacterial?

(Translation: *Do I need antibiotics?*)

The answer is challenging, because symptoms overlap, and although some rapid tests are available (for adenovirus, a common cause of viral conjunctivitis), these point-of-care tests are not commonly used for a variety of reasons, including current pricing and insurance reimbursement. **Current standard of care (for adult, non-contact lens wearers) is to hold off on antibiotic drops unless symptoms have persisted for more than one to two days, because even most bacterial infections are self-limited.**

Something you never wanted to know:

Sexually transmitted bacterial infections (STIs) like chlamydia and gonorrhea can end up in your eye directly from infected body fluids, especially if you performed oral sex on your partner or from touching your eye with a hand that has touched those fluids.

- **Chlamydia** is often isolated to one eye, and symptoms may persist for weeks. Clinicians often only discover this when other treatment has failed, at which point additional testing reveals chlamydia. Oral antibiotics are required to cure this infection.
- **Gonorrhea** is fortunately less common and tends to have profuse yellow-green discharge that sticks your eyelids together. Untreated, this serious infection can progress to potentially lethal sepsis and meningitis. Due to rapidly emerging drug resistance, all gonorrheal infections must be treated with both oral and injectable antibiotics (in addition to prescription eyedrops for gonorrheal eye infection).
- **Herpes Simplex** is a viral STI than can show up in your eye, often transmitted from a mouth sore to the eye from sequentially touching your mouth and eye, or from wetting a contact by putting it in your mouth—so **please** don't do that! Herpes eye infections tend to be quite painful and can rapidly progress to a very serious, potentially blinding infection.
- **All three** of these infections can be passed from an infected mother to her newborn's eyes during delivery.
- See Chapter 45: Sexually Transmitted Infections (Yes, It Happens to People like You), page 221.

Head to your doctor:
- **If you wear contacts** and have ANY type of pink eye or eye pain.
- If you have heavy eye discharge, pain, light sensitivity, or change in vision.

Worst-case scenario:
Bacterial eye infections, especially in people who wear contacts, can progress to more serious cornea infections, scarring the cornea and even causing blindness.

Prevention:
- Good hand washing and avoiding touching your mouth, nose, and eyes.

- Barrier use (condoms) for all sexual intimacy, including oral sex (yes, that's why flavored condoms were invented)
- NEVER share mascara or eye liner.
- NEVER sleep with your contacts in.

TIPS:

o **If you start having irritated, itchy, red eyes,** immediately remove your contacts and start using an OTC moisturizing drop such as artificial tears, Systane, or Blink.
  o Do *not* use the "get the red out" ones—these only temporarily shrink the blood vessels, "removing" the red. Overuse of these products is very common and will lead to dependence and chronic eye irritation.
o **If diagnosed with infectious "pink eye":**
  o **Throw away** your current contacts and any mascara!
  o **Wear your prescription glasses for a whole week** (or until your eye symptoms have been completely resolved for a couple days). While you have symptoms, *wear your glasses all the time* to keep you from touching your eyes involuntarily, even if you feel you don't fully need them.
  o **Wash your pillow sheet nightly** as long as you are having any eye discharge.
  o Please realize you are **contagious** for at least several days and up to a week, meaning ideally, do not go to class or meetings or work for a couple days. Your infection will not leap up and run across the room, but if you touch your eyes and then touch something else, you are leaving an infectious gift for the next person. Pay attention and especially avoid touching handrails, doorknobs, and other community property objects. Note that when your eyes are irritated, *it's really hard not to unintentionally touch your eyes!*
  o Carry **hand sanitizer** and use it early and often.

○ If you only have symptoms in one eye, **do not use eye drops in the other eye**, because you are likely to accidentally touch your infected eye with the bottle and then transmit that infection to your other eye.

○ Likewise, we know prescription drops are expensive, but please **do not save them** for your next bout of pink eye; you've likely introduced bacteria to the bottle.

Chapter 18
My Eye
(or Some Other Muscle)
Won't Stop Twitching

What If: My Eye (or Some Other Muscle) Won't Stop Twitching?

Medical Name: Myokymia (Eye Twitch) or Muscle Fasciculation

What most likely happened:

For the past week, you've been studying nonstop for midterms, pounding coffee to stay awake, and now your left lower eyelid (or section of your hand, forearm, eardrum, leg—really any isolated muscle) keeps twitching off and on throughout the day, driving you nuts.

What's going on?

The vast majority of the time, no direct metabolic explanation can be identified for a single twitching muscle. The nerve-muscle motor unit simply goes rogue, generating a rapid twitch of the muscle fibers. Dehydration, caffeine, nicotine, fatigue, and anxiety are all common potential triggers for this annoying symptom, especially when piled on top of one another. Electrolyte imbalances of sodium or potassium (from excess sweating, vomiting, or diarrhea), high or low calcium and magnesium, and excess lactic acid from muscle overexertion can also play a role. Twitches may also be a side effect from prescription medications such as antidepressants, antihistamines, stimulants (like ADHD meds or decongestants), and asthma medications.

Treatment:

Time. At the end of the day, we rarely find a treatable cause for twitches, and so we treat them by minimizing everything listed above that potentially can make them worse. Less caffeine, more rest, good hydration, and stress reduction are the mainstays of treatment. If we suspect the twitching is a medication side effect, your doctor may stop or change your prescriptions.

Head to your doctor:

If your muscle twitch lasts more than a few days, and especially if you begin experiencing multiple sites of muscle twitching, it's time for a clinician to examine you and possibly run some blood tests.

Worst-case scenario:

Typically, there is no worst case here! Dr. Google may warn of ALS (amyotrophic lateral sclerosis, a.k.a. Lou Gehrig's Disease), a progressive neurological disease that may indeed start with twitches. However, the roughly five thousand Americans diagnosed each year with this uncommon disease are typically much older than most college students (ages forty to seventy), their twitching is not limited to a single muscle, and they have multiple other symptoms like leg or arm weakness, slurred speech, and difficulty walking.

Prevention:

Especially when academic or emotional stresses pile up, focus on healthy habits and lifestyle choices:

- Exercise daily.
- Drink more water.
- Limit caffeine and alcohol.

- Make sure you aren't doubling up on stimulants (ADHD meds, decongestants, and caffeine) and LOOK FOR HIDDEN SOURCES OF CAFFEINE and other stimulants, like workout supplements and "natural" energy boost products.

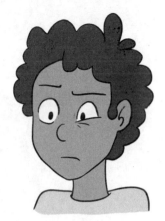

- Stop vaping.
- Sleep—consistent sleep and wake times, no all-nighters!

TIPS:

○ Don't stress over this one!

Chapter 19
Can't Hear?
Clogged Ear (Wax)

What If: My Ear Is Clogged (by Wax)?
Medical Name: Cerumen Impaction

What most likely happened:
For several days, you notice that you can't hear very well out of your right ear, even though you clean your ears every day with cotton swabs (like Q-tips). Now your ear is starting to hurt, especially when you use your ear buds. Wax buildup can cause fullness, pressure, pain, hearing loss, vertigo (feeling room spinning or off balance), or ringing in the affected ear.

What's going on?
- Ear wax (cerumen) is a normal substance produced and usually naturally extruded by the ear canal, typically asymptomatic (not noticed at all) in an estimated 95 percent of healthy adults.
- Netflix & Roommates! College students often wear ear buds with their smartphones or other electronic devices, or need to use earplugs to reduce roommate or dorm noise. Unfortunately, any device that sits in the ear canal can increase ear wax production and blockage.

- Using cotton swabs (or worse, bobby pins, please, **No!**) to "clean" your ears not only aggravates the problem but can cause damage to your ear canal or your eardrum.

Treatment:

Once wax has built up, dried up, and partially or fully blocked your ear canal, the treatment is removal by a clinician who can look inside your ear and visualize the eardrum (tympanic membrane). If the eardrum is intact, then options include irrigation (flushing out the ear with water) or manual removal (where the clinician uses a curette tool that looks like a metal stick with a small loop or tiny spoon on the end to gently pull out the wax).

Why does the physician get to use an object to remove the wax, but you should not? Because we can directly see where we are sticking that instrument and therefore can avoid damaging the canal or eardrum.

What about eardrops to remove wax? The medical term for these drops is "ceruminolytics," meaning that they break up the wax. However, the bottom line is that medical evidence is limited to support their effectiveness. Olive oil, vinegar, hydrogen peroxide, saline, water, and commercial products like Debrox all may help soften wax, but none of these should be used if there is an eardrum perforation (or surgically placed ear tubes) and therefore should not be used unless a clinician has looked in the ear and can verify the eardrum is intact. In my clinical practice, I have found little benefit from these agents in the college-age population.

Head to your doctor if:

With ear wax, there is no fever or visible swelling or redness to tell you when to be seen, so basically if you are having isolated ear discomfort, muffled hearing, ringing in your ears, or feeling off balance along with ear pressure, it's time to get checked out.

If, however, you are having mild ear symptoms along with allergy symptoms such as runny nose and sneezing, it's reasonable to try some over-the-counter antihistamine and decongestant combos for a day or two first, but if not improving, head on in.

Worst-case scenario:

You decide to use a bobby pin or cotton swab to remove the wax yourself, because you've always done that and never had a problem, but this time you accidentally rupture your eardrum. Trust me, this happens ALL THE TIME! Either you dig deeper "one last time" because you've almost got the wax out, or someone startles or bumps into you, causing you to accidentally thrust deeper. Now you have super sharp pain and possibly blood or blood-stained wax coming out of your ear. Head straight over to the clinic to be seen! Most ruptures can be treated with medications and manual removal of wax, but some are severe enough that they require surgical repair by a specialist.

Prevention:

- If you are a wax-builder-upper, flushing your ears out with lukewarm water once every four to eight weeks often avoids needing to go in to the doctor for removal.
- Stop using Q-tips (or anything else) to clean inside your ear canal.

TIPS:

- O **Never** stick anything inside your ear canal to "clean" your ear—no fingers, bobby pins, cotton-tipped applicators, or anything else!
- O Odds are good that if you do use cotton swabs, your ear problem (trauma to the canal, eardrum, or simply packed-hard wax) will be on your dominant-handed side, because that's the side where you maneuver best and have more force.
- O If your doctor has suggested you flush your ear to remove wax, use a baby nasal syringe (a plastic bulb) with lukewarm water (hot or cold water will make you feel very dizzy). Gently pull the ear upward and back (to straighten the canal), leaning over the sink with your head turned so the ear you will flush is facing the sink, and then barely insert the tip of the bulb in the canal and squeeze the bulb to flush the ear. Repeat this several times until you see wax floating out, no more than six to eight times per ear. Not working after a couple days? Head back to your doctor.

Chapter 20
Is This an Ear Infection?

What If: My Ear Is Clogged and Hurting (a.k.a. Do I Have an Ear Infection?)

Medical Name: Eustachian Tube Dysfunction, Otitis Media, & Otitis Externa

What most likely happened:

Scenario A: You began with a sore or scratchy throat and stuffy nose, and now one ear is stopped up and won't clear. Along with feeling full, plugged up, and uncomfortable or frankly even painful, you may notice trouble hearing or develop ringing in that ear, plus or minus fever.

Scenario B: During your flight back to school, your ears hurt a bit during take-off, then despite chewing gum during landing, your ears hurt even worse, and since then, you can't clear one of your ears.

Scenario C: You went scuba diving or, more commonly, you simply dove into the deep end of a pool to retrieve something from the bottom; and while still in the water, one or both of your ears developed intense pain.

Scenario D: You haven't been sick or had allergies, no recent fun beach trips, nothing out of the ordinary, but for no obvious reason, one ear starts to hurt.

109

What's going on?

The common cold, seasonal allergies, and sinus infections all can produce excess mucus and inflammation within the tubes (Eustachian tubes) that connect your middle ear (the area behind your eardrum) to the back of your nose and throat. These tubes typically remain closed unless you swallow, yawn, or chew, so that "clearing," crackly noise you hear in healthy ears when you do any of those activities is actually the sound of air moving as your tubes temporarily open. When this tube is blocked with mucus or swelling, a negative pressure is created that sucks your eardrum backward, causing ear pain through the eardrum's excellent nerve supply. Additionally, the blocked and often mucus-filled tube is fertile ground for any respiratory virus or bacteria, so infection may set in if the Eustachian tubes won't clear.

With flying, as the plane takes off and flies upward, the cabin air pressure drops, creating a positive pressure within the Eustachian tube that pushes forward on the eardrum. During landing, the air pressure is steadily increasing, creating negative pressure that sucks the eardrum backward as the tube closes. Healthy Eustachian tubes handle this by popping back open as you swallow; however, swollen or mucus-blocked tubes may get stuck closed. If this happens, you may need multiple interventions and significantly more time to reopen the tube and relieve your pain.

Any altitude change can cause ear "clogging" and pressure, especially if you already have allergies or a cold, including less dramatic height changes like riding elevators or driving up and down through hills.

Diving causes the same problems in reverse, with external water pressure building as you descend into the water, pushing back on the eardrum and causing a "squeeze." If the Eustachian tube cannot equalize, the eardrum can rupture, allowing cold ocean water to enter the ear and cause acute nausea, dizziness, and hearing loss.

Last, while the above issues all exist within the inner or middle ear, "swimmer's ear" affects only the **outer** portion of the ear. Prolonged moisture from swimming or superficial scratches from ear buds, Q-tips, or fingers can break down the lining of the ear canal, allowing bacteria easier access to cause infection. Swimmer's ear may start with itchy ear canals but often mimics a ruptured eardrum, complete with swelling, pain, and discharge.

Treatment:
Self-treatment for "Clogged Ear":
- **Swallow** as much as possible
  - Drink any beverage.
  - Chew gum.
  - Suck on sour candy (or anything that makes you salivate).
- **Yawn**
- **"Nose-Holding Pop":** *Only try this if you have no fever and no thick, discolored snot.*
  - Close your mouth and hold your nose, then gently blow.

OTC Medications for "Clogged Ear":
Although evidence is conflicting about efficacy, options include:
- Nasal steroid sprays (Flonase, Nasacort): slowly reduce swelling in the nasal membranes over several days
- Nasal decongestant sprays (Afrin): immediate, short-term shrinking of nasal membranes; do not use more than three days
- Oral decongestant pills (Sudafed)
- Antihistamines (Allegra/Claritin/Zyrtec/Benadryl)
- Nasal/sinus flushing with saline: neti pots

Prescription Medications:
Oral Antibiotics: Perhaps surprising news is that current medical evidence reveals that **many ear infections do *NOT* require antibiotics, even when they are bacterial, because most will resolve on their own.** As we work to limit antibiotic resistance (and see that even bacterial infections can usually resolve without antibiotics), doctors are holding off on antibiotics unless symptoms are severe (temperature greater than 101, intense pain) or symptoms are not improving after two to three days.

Topical Antibiotic Drops: With outer ear infections like swimmer's ear, or for middle ear infections when someone has a PE (Pressure Equalization) ear tube in place (and therefore direct access to the middle ear), antibiotic eardrops are the first-line prescription choice. If your doctor sees a ton of swelling inside your canal, they may choose an antibiotic drop that includes a steroid to decrease the inflammation.

Oral Steroids: Definitely not a first-line choice but may be added if needed, especially when seasonal allergies started your nasal and ear congestion.

Head to your doctor if you:

- Have severe ear pain; do **not** wait for a fever or ruptured eardrum!
- Cannot clear your ear despite trying above interventions for a day
- Develop ringing in your ears
- See any discharge or bleeding from your ear

Worst-case scenario:

If the pressure keeps building and there is no relief, the eardrum will rupture. If you have discharge or any blood coming out of your ear (often found on the pillow in the morning after a night of ear pain), please head to the doctor! With time (and usually antibiotics), a small rupture will usually repair itself, but occasionally the hole is large enough that it must be surgically repaired with a patch to preserve hearing.

For a Eustachian tube that refuses to open, doctors may opt to perform a tiny incision in the eardrum (called a myringotomy) to remove the built-up fluid from behind the eardrum. If this procedure is only temporarily successful, then a tiny plastic PE (Pressure Equalization) tube is surgically placed through the eardrum to maintain the opening longer. The tubes typically do not need to be removed, because the healing eardrum tissue slowly pushes them out as the tissue grows back in six to twelve months. Many college students do not know or remember if they had ear tubes as a toddler. However, if you remember needing custom earplugs to swim when you were little, then odds are good that you had tubes, and all that remains is a tiny scar on the eardrum that your doctor may note when she examines your ear.

Prevention:

- **Do not smoke or vape**: These fumes irritate your nasal and sinus membranes, creating inflammation and predisposing you to this problem.
- **If you have seasonal allergies:** Use nasal steroids daily during your allergen season.
- **Flights:** An hour or two before your flight, take an OTC decongestant like Sudafed. Bring a nasal decongestant spray (like Afrin) with you and use it right before you board the plane. Repeat the spray when you are about thirty minutes from landing. During both take-off and landing, plan to be actively swallowing by drinking water, sucking on candy, chewing gum, or yawning.

TIPS:

- To clear your ears, ***blowing up a balloon*** often works better than the "hold your nose and blow" method, but ONLY TRY THIS IF YOU DO NOT APPEAR INFECTED (no discolored, thick snot or fever).
- If you have one sore ear, try gently tugging on your ear lobe—if this makes it worse, you are more likely to have an outer ear infection like swimmer's ear, which typically requires treatment with prescription antibiotic drops.

Chapter 21
Ringing Ears

What If: My Ears Are Ringing?
Medical Name: Tinnitus

What most likely happened:

Scenario A: Last weekend's music festival rocked your world, complete with dancing for hours next to throbbing speakers . . . **or** you ended up with seats right next to the brass and percussion sections of the band at the football game yesterday . . . **or** you simply had to stay plugged in to your noise-cancelling ear buds in all night to drown out your suitemates' noise while you were studying and trying to get some sleep. In any case, upon awaking, you notice you've got ringing in one or both ears, which may make it difficult to hear clearly. You take a shower to clear your head, and then with blow-drying your hair, the ringing gets even louder.

Scenario B: You've had cold symptoms with nasal congestion and stopped-up ears for a few days, been taking combination cold remedies, and now your ears are ringing.

Scenario C: You've recently started vaping or smoking . . .

What's going on?

Ear ringing, called "tinnitus" in medical terms, is the perception of noise in the ears when there is no external noise. Some hear high-pitched whining, while others hear low buzzing sounds. Loud sounds from blaring music can damage fragile hair cells inside your ear, and then the brain misinterprets the messages from these injured areas as noise, or ringing. Although the most common cause of ear ringing is barotrauma (damage from loud noise), other causes include medication side effects (especially from aspirin), seasonal allergies, trauma to your head or ear, jaw problems, or stopped-up ears from either wax or congestion. Smoking or vaping makes you more likely to develop tinnitus (both directly and through the nasal and ear congestion caused from the vapors). Far less commonly in young adults, we may see the inner ear disease Meniere's (also has hearing loss and dizziness) or tinnitus caused by high blood pressure. *Very rarely*, the cause is a benign inner-ear tumor called an acoustic neuroma.

Treatment:

Often tinnitus will resolve quickly within hours or a day on its own, and no treatment is needed. However, with significant damage there can be partial hearing loss, and physicians may treat this condition with prescription oral steroids or other medications. Tinnitus does not always have an obvious cause, but a thorough evaluation will look for and try to treat or eliminate related issues like packed ear wax, dizziness, seasonal allergies, or medication side effects.

Head to your doctor if:
- Your ringing is increasing in volume.
- You have vertigo or hearing loss along with the ringing.
- You have sudden onset of ringing with no obvious cause.
- Your ringing is loud enough to bother and distract you.

Worst-case scenario:

Severe cases of tinnitus may not go away, particularly when there is associated hearing loss. Numerous interventions are available to help retrain the brain or mask the noise, as well as medications to reduce the severity of the symptoms, but chronic tinnitus is a very challenging problem.

Prevention:

- Protect your ears! Turn down the volume of your music and wear earplugs to concerts.
- If you are at a club with extremely loud music, take breaks and go outside with a friend.
- Don't smoke or vape.

TIPS:

- Use earplugs!! Seriously, **college students do use earplugs** for predictably loud situations—look at the band members at football and basketball games! No earplugs with you? Grab a napkin, tissue, or toilet paper and tear off a couple small sections that you can roll up and **gently** place in your ears.
- Invest in noise-cancelling earphones rather than cranking up the volume to drown out other noise around you.
- Take a short (five-to-ten-minute) break from your headphones every hour.
- Turn your volume down one "notch." Most of us listen to music or podcasts a bit louder than we need to in order to comfortably listen.

Chapter 22
Stuffy Nose, Colds, and Sinus Infections

What If: I Get Cold or Sinus Infection?
Medical Name: Upper Respiratory Infections and Acute Rhinosinusitis

What most likely happened:

Someone coughed or sneezed into the air near you or onto a high-touch surface (like a doorknob or handrail) shortly before you touched it, then you subsequently touched your own eyes, nose, or mouth and inadvertently welcomed their virus-containing respiratory droplets into your body. One or two days later, you develop classic cold symptoms: a stuffy and/or runny nose, mild sore throat, low-grade fever, headache, and an overall feeling of discomfort. *This is the common cold.*

Later that week, despite your symptoms steadily improving up until now, you start to develop new problems. Now the pain and pressure have settled in to one primary spot, usually along one side of your nose or forehead, and now your simple cold has leveled up to a sinus infection. If the infection is in one of the sinuses next to or behind your nose, aching upper teeth may be your primary frustration. Nasal secretions will thicken and discolor your snot to a lovely shade of yellow-green, and frankly, your breath could use a mint. Optional bonus features include fever, decreased

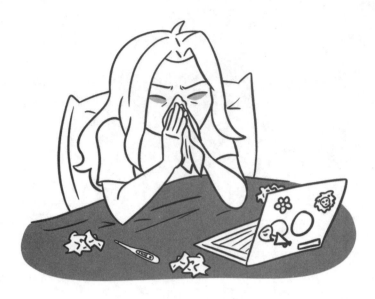

or altered sense of smell or taste, sore throat, hoarse voice (from the post-nasal drainage), and ear pain.

What's going on?

The common cold can be caused by a huge variety of respiratory viruses, with rhinovirus, respiratory syncytial virus (RSV), parainfluenza virus, adenovirus, and corona viruses (including but not limited to COVID-19) being the most common offenders. Cold symptoms are typically annoying but not incapacitating, so symptomatic treatment with over-the-counter decongestants and pain relievers will usually allow you to get through your normal tasks. The worst symptoms usually improve after a few days but other symptoms can linger for a week to ten days. *Antibiotics have no role in the treatment of these viral infections.*

The vast majority of acute sinus infections are also **VIRAL**; *only an estimated 0.5 to 2 percent are bacterial.* Sinuses are simply hollowed-out sections of the facial bones, and when inflammation fills these structures with mucus, they become a homemade culture plate for infection. An acute sinusitis may last up to four weeks, while chronic sinusitis exceeds three months. Chronic sinusitis may involve a persistent infection, but more commonly this condition evolves from a prolonged inflammatory response clogging up your nasal passages and sinuses.

Treatment:

Since virtually all colds and the vast majority of sinus infections are viral, *antibiotics are rarely indicated.*

Treatment is therefore aimed at symptomatic relief to ease nasal congestion, headaches, body aches, sore throats, and coughs.

Staying "well-hydrated" helps you feel better with all respiratory infections because your fever and faster breathing work to dehydrate you, which makes head and body aches worse and makes your mucus drier and stickier, tougher to clear.

- Don't chug (because that often makes people throw up, especially if they have heavy post-nasal mucus drainage); instead, steadily sip enough liquid that you need to pee at least every few hours.
- What liquid is best? The one you will drink! Choose or alternate water, electrolyte replacement drinks (Pedialyte, Ultima Replenisher, Liquid IV, etc.), or sport drinks (Gatorade, Powerade, Propel, etc.)

Rest
- Hang out in your bed, couch, or chair, but take screen breaks and actually SLEEP.

Isolate to avoid spreading your respiratory infection to others.
- **How long?** Talk with your doctor, but at least until you are feeling better, and you've had NO FEVER for twenty-four hours WITHOUT using any fever-lowering medications like acetaminophen (Tylenol) or ibuprofen (Advil).
- As of 2024, the recommendation for COVID isolation time is five days.

Current clinical practice guidelines only recommend:
- Nasal saline washes*
- OTC nasal steroid sprays to decrease inflammation
- OTC pain relievers such as Tylenol or ibuprofen (Advil)

*Nasal saline wash recommendations:
- Talk with your doctor if you want to make your own solution.
- Never use tap water without first boiling for several minutes and completely cooling; generally, distilled water is preferred (if making your own solution) or simply purchase sterile saline or another product your doctor recommends.
- Low pressure, high-volume flushing (~240cc) works better than nasal saline sprays.
- Hypertonic saline (more salt) may be more irritating than isotonic (less salt) solutions; efficacy of one versus the other is inconsistent.
- Devices such as neti pots work well, but be certain to cleanse regularly and air dry completely after each use.
- Frequency? Once daily to a few times per week.

*"But my mom, a friend, a commercial, or Dr. Google said these help (even though they are **not** backed by scientific studies). Should I try . . . ?"*

- **Decongestants:** Maybe, especially if you have ear pressure/ pain. Oral pills like Sudafed* or topical sprays like Afrin may help nasal stuffiness or ear pressure (see Chapter 20: Is This an Ear Infection?, page 109), but only use for a maximum of three days because otherwise they backfire, causing worsening of your symptoms through rebound swelling.

  * By federal standards, pseudoephedrine (Sudafed) does not require a prescription, but all sales are documented "behind the counter" because of the potential abuse of this product to manufacture illegal methamphetamine; specific restrictions vary by state. The bottom line is that you will need to go to the pharmacy counter and ask for this medication because

it will not be sitting out on the shelves. Easily accessed over-the-counter decongestants currently include phenylephrine (including OTC Sudafed PE) but with the September 2023 FDA Advisory Committee's announcement showing current doses of oral phenylephrine are ineffective (although not harmful) as a decongestant, these products are no longer recommended and may be removed.

- **Expectorants:** Designed to break up mucus; sounds helpful, so we prescribed these for years, but turns out there's no good evidence that they speed healing or help symptoms.
- **Antihistamines:** *Not helpful* in infectious sinusitis.
    - Why not? Antihistamines are too drying, and side effects outweigh benefits; they create thinner but sticky mucus, less able to clear out of the sinus.

What about OTC Supplements?

- Vitamin D
    - People with low Vitamin D levels have an increased risk of respiratory infections, whether the cause is a common cold, influenza, or COVID. Taking Vitamin D if you have normal blood levels of this vitamin may not be helpful, but when taken at levels between the recommended daily amount of 600IU and the recommended upper limit of 4000IU/day, it should not be harmful.
- Zinc
    - Zinc lozenges (that you suck on, not pills that you swallow) have been shown in some studies to reduce the duration of the common cold by roughly one day. Using zinc lozenges at or below the recommended upper limit dose of 40mg/day should not cause harm. Note: Zinc lozenges can result in a distinctive metallic taste that can be confused with the altered taste associated with COVID infection.

- NEVER use Zinc NASAL SPRAYS, as they can cause permanent loss of smell.
- Vitamin C
  - Vitamin C is a perennial favorite for colds and other upper respiratory viruses, although evidence is at best, conflicting. Consuming less than the recommended upper limit of 2000mg (including food sources and your supplement) is usually not harmful. However, exceeding 2000mg per day can cause gastrointestinal upset (heartburn, gastritis, nausea, vomiting or diarrhea), headaches, insomnia, and even kidney stones. The actual recommended daily allowance is 75 to 100mg.

Do I need an X-ray? *No, not for a typical acute sinus infection.* Sinus X-rays and CT scans are only indicated for long, persisting symptoms (usually more than three months) or complications.

Head to your doctor if:
- Pain becomes severe.
- You have trouble breathing.
- Your vision is affected (blurry or double vision).
- Bending your neck hurts (stiff neck).
- You become confused or mentally sluggish.
- Fever persists beyond a day or two.
- You have blisters, swelling, or redness anywhere on your face.
- Symptoms last more than a week.

Worst-case scenario:

The worst case for a "cold" is developing a severe COVID infection that requires hospitalization or developing "long COVID" symptoms that can include symptoms such as brain fog, mental health concerns, breathing difficulty, headaches, fatigue, and cardiovascular problems. The very rare but worst case for an acute sinusitis would be the infection extending locally into the eyes, skull bones, or brain (meningitis), any of which can be life-threatening.

More commonly, the worst case is developing chronic or recurrent sinusitis that may ultimately require surgery to physically enlarge your natural drainage pathways and remove obstructions that have developed (like nasal polyps).

Prevention:

Hand Washing! This is always the best way to help prevent respiratory infections. Remember this is not a two-second pass under the bathroom faucet, but a full twenty seconds of scrubbing the top, bottom, and sides of your hands with soap or sanitizer.

If you have seasonal allergies, talk with your doctor about using a daily nasal steroid spray to reduce swelling and obstruction in your nasal passages.

Vaccinate: The annual flu vaccine certainly will not prevent common colds, but it will decrease the severity of your flu symptoms if you become infected. Similarly, although most COVID infections are mild in the healthy college student population, COVID vaccines remain our best defense against severe disease, hospitalization, and death (especially for those at higher risk.)

A Few Thoughts about COVID

When the COVID pandemic began in the spring of 2020, infections seemed unstoppable, as did the deaths. The world abruptly stopped, rearranging life around this dangerous respiratory virus that overwhelmed our hospitals and clogged our ICUs. Today, immunity from previous infections and vaccinations has helped the world stagger toward normalcy. COVID is now considered an endemic virus, meaning it is constantly present at a baseline level and we must learn to live with it. If we are too afraid of the virus, we might end up losing out on too much. If we ignore the reality of COVID and other respiratory viruses, that can cost us, too. Pranay Sinha, MD, an assistant professor of medicine in infectious disease at Boston University Chobanian & Avedisian School of Medicine, suggests a pragmatic harm-reduction approach with these three tips:

1. **Prioritize activities:** Perhaps you have something fun coming up, like a nonrefundable spring break trip to Europe; or less fun, like a huge paper or a major exam; or maybe you're going to spend a holiday with older relatives or someone with a weakened immune system. These are situations where you can't afford to be ill, either for your own sake or for the sake of others. ***Play it extra-safe the week beforehand.*** Avoid dense crowds, choose outdoor barbecues rather than crowded bars, wear masks on the subway, order in instead of eating out. At other times, you may not need to be as limited.

2. **Develop situational awareness**: Keep an eye on COVID like you would on the weather. If news reports tell you COVID hospitalization rates are rising, start thinking about how that may affect you and, again, ramp up your caution.

3. **Safeguard others**: Despite your best efforts, you may get infected or even re-infected with COVID. If this happens, be kind to yourself, but also please be considerate of others. Try to get tested early, isolate from others, and focus on getting better. Your goal should be to *let the spread end with you*. PS: This is also true for any other infectious disease!

TIPS:

- **Green snot does not equal need for antibiotics!** Remember **most** sinus infections are **viral**, so antibiotics do not help.
- **Antihistamines do NOT help** sinus infections and often make them worse.
- If your breath is awful and your upper teeth ache on the same side as your stuffy nose (made worse with bending forward or tapping on your face where it hurts), these are clues that you may have developed a bacterial sinus infection.
- Avoid "high-touch" surfaces like handrails and doorknobs, and/or carry some hand sanitizer with you to use routinely for a full twenty-second cleanse.
- Avoid sharing drinks and makeup (especially lip products); these are high-speed transit for germs.

Chapter 23
Nose Bleeds

What If: I Get Nosebleeds (Without Being Hit in the Nose)?

Medical name: Epistasis

What most likely happened:

Cold outside temperatures create superdry air inside from constant heaters (or in the South, we see this vice versa with universal air conditioning during the summer). On your way to class, you briefly pick your nose because it feels like something is there . . . and suddenly you've got blood dripping down your face. (This is SO embarrassing, but it happens quite often.) Or sometimes nosebleeds are purely spontaneous, so you reach up to wipe what you think is a dripping runny nose and discover blood instead.

What's going on?

"Digital trauma"—the number-one cause of nosebleeds is picking your nose. *No other way to say it.* ¯_(ツ)_/¯

- Dry nasal membranes bleed very easily with minimal disturbance
  - Medications are often to blame for the dryness
    - Antihistamines (allergy meds like Allegra, Claritin, Zyrtec)

- - Antidepressant or antianxiety meds
  - Environment (indoor A/C or heat)
- Seasonal allergies or sinus infections
- Smoking (or vaping) directly irritates your nasal membranes, making them more fragile and likely to bleed
- Snorting cocaine (or sniffing glue, and obviously any other substance you put up your nose)
- Blood thinners (like aspirin) make you bleed more easily everywhere, including your nose.

Treatment:

- Stand or preferably sit up, leaning a bit forward (to keep blood going out your nose, not down your throat).
- **Pressure**—Use your thumb and index finger to hold firm pressure above the nostrils but below the nasal bones and do **not** let go to "check" on the bleed for at least ten minutes.
- If you have ice handy, add an ice pack on top of your nose but do **not** let go of pinching to do this.
- **Then** gently blow out any clotted blood and consider administering one spray in the bleeding nostril of a nasal decongestant like Afrin (oxymetazoline) and hold pressure again for another five to ten minutes.

Head to your doctor if:

- **One-time nosebleed?** Embarrassing, but no big deal . . . unless you can't get it to stop bleeding within fifteen to twenty minutes with holding direct pressure. Have someone take you to your doctor if you can't make the bleeding stop (while you keep holding pressure).
- **Nosebleeds happening several times in one week?** Time for a visit to look for an underlying cause.

Worst-case scenario:

Ninety percent of nosebleeds come from the front portion of the nose, and the vast majority can be controlled with direct pressure and topical spray medication. Rarely, these anterior bleeds require additional intervention, most commonly a clinician applying silver nitrate to chemically cauterize the blood vessels or placing packing inside the nose (which is well within the scope of most campus clinics). However, especially with the 10 percent of nosebleeds that occur in the posterior portion of the nose, bleeding can be severe enough to require hospitalization and even surgical repair under anesthesia.

Prevention:

- Try to not pick your nose.
- Stay hydrated by drinking more water and limiting caffeine.
- Dry air? Use a humidifier in your room.
- For seasonal allergies, consider using daily nasal steroid sprays (to help reduce how often you need oral antihistamines).
- Consider nasal saline washes if you have chronic sinus issues.
- Stop smoking/vaping/putting any toxic substance in your nose.

TIPS:

- If you have an extremely heavy, rapid nose bleed, the blood can literally back up through your tear ducts, and blood will flow into your eyes and out on your face as bloody "tears." This occurs infrequently but is hugely dramatic for anyone witnessing; however, simply treat this nosebleed like any other.
- If you've held pressure constantly for ten minutes but still have bleeding, try one squirt of Afrin in your bleeding nostril and hold pressure another five minutes before heading to your doctor.

Chapter 24

Itching, Sneezing, Allergies, and Hives

What If: I'm Itching, Sneezing, Having Allergies, or Getting Hives?

Medical Name: Allergic Rhinitis, Allergic Conjunctivitis, or Urticaria

What most likely happened:

Scenario A: You've moved across the country (or even across the state), and now new irritants from local trees, grasses, ragweed, or molds are giving you itchy eyes, runny nose, sneezing, and/or a scratchy-turned-really-sore throat . . . except since you've never had allergies before, you're convinced you've got a cold that won't go away. Taking diphenhydramine (Benadryl) at bedtime helps you sleep but leaves you with morning brain fog and dry mouth.

Scenario B: The itching began right after your hot shower this morning, progressively worsening during your first lecture, and now hives are erupting on your neck, arms, and legs. You didn't feel anything sting you and haven't eaten anything unusual, so what else could this be?

What's going on?

A. Allergens like pollen come in contact with your eyes and nose; your body interprets these substances as harmful and sends out the troops via an inflammatory response. Part of that response includes releasing chemicals like histamine, which in turn increases local blood flow, stimulates mucus production, and makes you itch. Eyes become bloodshot and itchy, often with a slight stringy discharge (see Chapter 17: Pink Eye: Infectious or Allergic?, page 96). Your nose and sinuses feel stuffy or drippy, which may create pressure in your ears or cause pain in your throat from postnasal drainage.

 B. Histamine release in the skin can cause itching and hives, which are transient, raised, red swollen areas with well-defined borders. Sometimes they merge together, and typically clusters of them come and go. Hives themselves are easy to recognize and reasonably straightforward to treat, but identifying their cause can be challenging or impossible. Seasonal allergens, foods, medications, perfumes, shampoo, lotions, laundry detergents, preservatives, and insect bites or stings can all trigger hives; and to complicate things further, you can react to something the first or the hundredth time you are exposed to it, so the fact that you've never had a problem eating mango before does not mean the mango you ate today didn't trigger your hives.

Treatment:

- **Nasal steroid sprays:** Fluticasone (Flonase), triamcinolone (Nasacort), etc. Previously prescription, now several are OTC; they're not "pump-you-up" steroids, but anti-inflammatory, acting locally in your nose and sinuses to decrease inflammation and prevent the allergic response before it begins.
- **Oral Antihistamine Medications:** These medications can't stop the inflammatory process in progress, but they can shut down additional release of histamine. These are first-line treatments for hives.

- Sedating: Diphenhydramine (Benadryl) or chlorpheniramine (Chlor-Trimeton), dimenhydrinate (Dramamine)
  - Nonsedating: Fexofenadine (Allegra), loratadine (Claritin), cetirizine (Zyrtec)
- **Steroids**:
  - Topical products (creams, ointments, and gels)
    - OTC hydrocortisone
    - Stronger prescription steroids
  - Oral steroids (prednisone and depomedrol, often in "dose packs")
  - Injectable steroids (typically given as a shot in your hip)

Head to your doctor if:
- OTC medications are not helping.
- You develop fever (temp is greater than 100.5).
- You have any shortness of breath or trouble swallowing.
- You start having nose bleeds.

Worst-case scenario:
Any type of allergic reaction can flare into an anaphylactic reaction that can literally take your breath away. If you develop swelling in your lips, trouble swallowing, tightness in your chest, cough, or shortness of breath, tell someone and seek help immediately. Anaphylaxis requires trained medical interventions (with epinephrine, IV fluids, and airway support).

Prevention:
- Daily nasal steroid sprays are the best OTC prevention for seasonal allergies.
- For allergic symptoms resistant to OTC and prescription medications, consider seeing an Allergy/Immunology physician for specific allergy skin or blood testing and desensitization allergy shots.

- Montelukast (Singulair) is a prescription oral medication that can be taken daily to limit your body's overactive inflammatory response to allergens; this is typically a second-line drug used when nasal steroids and oral antihistamines are not working or have unacceptable side effects.

TIPS:

o Some of the most painful sore throats are "just" allergies!
   o *Degree of pain does not determine allergy versus infection.*
o When using a nasal steroid spray, blow your nose first, then aim the spray straight toward the back of your head (avoiding the septum). Keep the spray next to your toothbrush so you remember to use it every day, because these take several days to a week to become fully effective. Use nasal steroids **daily** (during your "season") and add oral antihistamines as needed (rather than vice versa). Which OTC nasal steroid is best, Flonase, Nasacort, or a generic of either? Flonase has a distinctive floral smell that some people prefer and others dislike, but otherwise, studies show they are all equivalent. Grab whichever one you will use consistently!
o Saline sinus flushes like the neti pot may help with nasal congestion.
   o See Chapter 22: Stuffy Nose, Colds, and Sinus Infections (page 117).
o Heat releases histamine, so **hot showers are going to make you itch more**, whatever the cause. Shower with **cool** water if you are itchy or have hives.
o If you use a hypoallergenic laundry detergent (like Tide Free & Gentle or All Free & Clear) but have to use a shared community washer and dryer, know you are still exposed to allergens from other people's detergents. Some dorms and apartments will designate at least one set of washer/dryers as hypoallergenic. ASK for this if yours does not do that yet.

O   Do **not** use OTC "get the red out" eye drops (like Visine) or
    "immediate relief" nasal congestion sprays (like Afrin) more than
    three days; these products constrict the blood vessels in your
    eyes/nose, respectively, and give temporary relief but can lead to
    dependence and rebound congestion.

Chapter 25
Cold Sores and Fever Blisters

What If: I Get a Cold Sore/Fever Blister?

Medical Name: Herpes Simplex Virus

What most likely happened:

The last few days, you noticed a couple small red bumps off the side of your upper lip, barely above the top edge. "Great, more pimples," you assume. But today the bumps are multiplying, merging, hurting, turning red, and starting to blister. Your roommate, who gets cold sores all the time, tosses a tube of cream to you, saying, "Here, use this for your fever blister." What? You've never had a fever blister before.

What's going on?

Herpes Simplex Virus (**HSV**, not to be confused with **HIV**) causes recurrent outbreaks of small clusters of painful bumps that first blister and then crust over, commonly referred to as "cold sores" or "fever blisters." This virus is spread by direct skin-to-skin contact from another person and infects one area on your body (either your mouth or genitals). After the blisters scab up and disappear, the herpes virus goes into remission, hanging out in the nervous system until some physical, emotional, or immune-related stressor triggers the virus to erupt again in the same general area. The frequency of recurrent eruptions or "outbreaks" varies greatly from person to person, from none to multiple times per year.

Oral HSV is EXTREMELY COMMON, with blood antibody tests showing that nearly half (47.8 percent) of the adult population in the United States (and 67 percent of the global population) are affected, although many of these people are unaware, because they are not bothered by any symptoms. Many people are infected from nonsexual close contact with family or friends, by kissing or sharing utensils, drinks, or lip products. *The infection can be passed from one person to another whether or not the infected individual has a visible blister*. Yes, herpes is **most** contagious when you have an active blister (and the couple days immediately before and right after the blister), but the virus also "sheds" sporadically on other days even when there are no blisters.

Herpes simplex virus comes in two "flavors"—HSV type 1 and HSV type 2. The vast majority of oral herpes infections (cold sores) are type 1. Both types produce similar-looking lesions, and BOTH can be transmitted via oral/genital contact (a.k.a. oral sex). Let's be clear, this can work in either direction, mouth to genitals or genitals to mouth, though it's far more common to see transmission from mouths to genitals. *In fact, over half of **new** genital herpes cases are the result of receiving oral sex from a partner who has HSV type 1.* The good news, however, is that genital herpes that is type 1 (from your partner's "cold sore" mouth infection) is far less likely to have **recurrent** breakouts and, happily, also less likely to be passed on to future partners.

Treatment:

Although we do not have any medications yet that will permanently eradicate HSV and leave you "cured," we have plenty of antiviral medications that reduce the severity and duration of infection. These same medications can also be used to prevent outbreaks or prevent spread of infection to a partner.

- Topical medications (safe but not dramatically more effective than placebo)
  - Prescription Antiviral: Acyclovir ointment (Denavir)

- Nonprescription but FDA approved antiviral: Abreva
- Prescription oral antiviral medications: Acyclovir (Zovirax), Valacyclovir (Valtrex), and Famciclovir (Famvir)
- Herbal: Mostly lysine, but buyer beware—*scientific evidence is conflicting at best.*

Head to your doctor if:
- You have never had a fever blister before, so let's be sure about your diagnosis **and** make sure all your questions are answered!
- Your symptoms are severe, especially if you are also having fever, swollen neck glands, and/or lesions in your mouth that make eating or drinking painful.
- You begin having recurrent outbreaks.
- You develop any eye discomfort.

Worst-case scenario:
Especially during an *initial* infection with HSV, accidentally touching your eye immediately after touching your blisters can directly spread that infection to your eye. HSV eye infections are potentially very serious and painful; immediate referral to an ophthalmologist is mandatory.

More commonly, the worst-case scenario is passing your simple "cold sore" to a new sexual partner via oral sex, giving them genital herpes because you were too embarrassed/shy/whatever to talk about and use a barrier.

- See Chapter 45: Sexually Transmitted Infections (Yes, It Happens to People like You) on page 221.

Prevention:
- Avoid sharing lip products (gloss, Chap Stick), drinks, or eating utensils.
- **Sunlight** is a consistent trigger for outbreaks, especially after a day of snow skiing or beach/water activity, so block that sun with SPF 30 sunscreen lip balm and/or a hat.

- If you have an HSV prescription for outbreaks, talk to your doctor about how to take it preventatively (typically once daily) for known triggers (think Spring Break in Cancun).
- Use a **barrier** if you are giving or receiving oral sex (condom or dental dam).

TIPS:

○ Don't confuse **canker** sores (aphthous ulcers) with HSV. Canker sores are the most common sores inside mouths—typically tiny, painful white sores on the tongue or inner surface of the lips, lasting around a week. Canker sores are **not** contagious; causes include microtrauma from brushing teeth, acidic food, smoking/vaping, stress, etc.

○ If this is your first cold sore and you wear **contacts**, switch to glasses until your symptoms have resolved to minimize the risk of accidentally spreading the infection. *We absentmindedly touch our mouths, nose, and eyes far more often than you realize.*

○ For recurrent cold sores, pay attention to triggers and early symptoms (tingling or burning **before** you see blisters in the area where you typically break out), because the sooner you start antiviral medications, the better they work to prevent or heal an outbreak.

Chapter 26
Bad Breath
and Tonsil Stones

What If: I Get Bad Breath?
Medical name: Halitosis & Tonsilloliths

What most likely happened:
Sometimes your breath is so yucky, you can smell it or taste it yourself, but often this embarrassing news comes from a significant other, BFF, or room-mate. Pay attention if your close friends are constantly offering you breath mints! Seriously, if friends can't tell each other about bad breath, well, who can? Obviously, foods like onions or garlic can cause temporary bad breath, but that's nothing a few mints, mouthwash, and brushing your teeth won't handle. Here we're talking about being "that" person with bad breath.

What's going on?
- **Dehydration:** The mouth needs to stay moist (making saliva) to keep your mouth clean. *Antihistamines and other meds are common culprits of dry mouth.*
- **Postnasal drainage**: Mucus dripping down the back of your throat, typically worse in the morning, is another very common

cause. Seasonal allergies, sinus infections, or respiratory viruses like the common cold all cause this.

- **Tonsilloliths:** If you are looking in the back of your mouth and you see (or cough/gag/spit up) a pea-sized, whitish-to-light-yellow, cheesy-consistency, foul-smelling ball stuck in/on your tonsil, **that** is a tonsil stone, definitely a source of bad breath. Tonsilloliths occur when tiny pieces of food get stuck in the folds/crypts of your tonsil tissue, and then bacteria, dead cells, and inflammatory cells combine to create these layered and often calcified "rocks."

- **Smoking/vaping**: Duh. The smoky vapor stains and irritates your teeth, tongue, and gums, plus provides the added benefit of ashtray breath.

- **Poor dental hygiene**: Again, you know this. If you don't brush your teeth and gums regularly (plus, ideally, floss), tiny bits of food get left behind, basically rotting as the bacteria in your mouth break it down. Gross.

- **Extreme dieting:** Diets that are low carb/low calorie such as Atkins or Keto create bad breath from the ketones your body creates when it is breaking down fat (instead of carbs) for fuel.

Treatment:

Varies by **cause**:

- **Dehydration**: Drink more water, cut back on caffeine (because it's a diuretic—makes you more dehydrated), and check your medications to see if they are making things worse. Common meds that cause dry mouth: antihistamines (Benadryl, Allegra, Zyrtec, Claritin), sleep aids (mostly contain Benadryl/diphenhydramine), ADHD medications (Adderall, Vyvanse, etc.), and antidepressant/antianxiety meds.

- **Postnasal drainage:** If you have seasonal allergies, consider starting an OTC daily nasal steroid spray, noting that antihistamine pills can aggravate bad breath because of dehydration. If you think the drainage is from a sinus or respiratory infection, treat accordingly.

- **Tonsilloliths:** Frustratingly, there is no easy fix. Improving dental hygiene, gargles, manual removal, and antibiotics may all be utilized.
- **Smoking/vaping:** Yet another reason to **Quit Smoking!** If you can't quit yet, know you have to be at least twice as diligent about dental hygiene.
- **Poor dental hygiene:** Brush your teeth, gums, **and** tongue at least twice per day, making sure to brush right before you go to bed. Flossing is critical—there's no way around it. Try to floss once each day. Mouthwash after you brush and floss. Talk with your dentist or dental hygienist to be sure you understand the right techniques to brush; most people do it wrong (not brushing long enough or brushing way too hard or too soft).
- **Keto-inducing diets:** The only way to stop the keto breath is to introduce more carbs; often going low-carb instead of no-carb does the trick. (And, of course, we need vegetables and fruits in our diets for balanced nutrition.)

Head to your doctor if:
- You are worried about having bad breath.
- You see "stuff" on your tonsils—pus or what you believe to be tonsil stones.
- You would like help quitting smoking or vaping.

Worst-case scenario:

Very rarely, tonsil stones will recur so frequently or be so troublesome that doctors will recommend surgically removing your tonsils.

Prevention:
- Consistent attention to your routine dental hygiene:
  - Brush your teeth for a full two minutes, twice per day.
  - Floss daily.
- See your dentist every six months.
- Never smoke/vape.

TIPS:

- ○ If your **toothbrush bristles are splayed out**, you are *brushing too hard* and it's time to **replace your toothbrush**. Use soft, circular motions to brush.

- ○ Invest in a high-quality electric toothbrush like Sonicare or Oral B and USE it twice every day, for a full two minutes each time. Pro tip: Play your favorite two-minute songs to push you to go the full time! Dentists and dental hygienists swear that making this one change will whiten your teeth, improve your breath, and shorten your time in their dental chair.

- ○ Thinking about mirror-assisted self-surgery and using a toothpick to dig out that tonsil stone? You've probably already tried, but seriously, **stop**! Take a hard pass on this one, because tonsils love to bleed and/or get infected when we muck around back there. You do *not* want your next surgery to be an emergency tonsillectomy!

Chapter 27

When Your Sore Throat Is Strep

What If: I Have a Bad Sore Throat (Is It Strep?)

Medical name: Strep Pharyngitis

What most likely happened:

You felt completely fine the last several days, but after your last class yesterday, you noticed a moderate sore throat that steadily got worse while you studied. Trying to avoid getting sick, you popped a couple ibuprofen tablets and went to bed early around 10:00 p.m. You a woke from a fitful sleep around 3:00 a.m. because the ibuprofen had 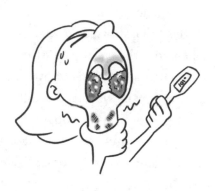 worn off, and merely swallowing saliva felt like you have razor blades in your throat. Your T-shirt was soaked with sweat, your face flushed, and it felt like you had a fever . . . confirmed to be 101.4°F by the thermometer that your mom thoughtfully included in your first aid kit. By morning, the glands in the front of your throat felt swollen and tender to touch, but you had no runny nose, no cough—nothing else except your ridiculously

141

painful throat. Looking in the mirror and using your iPhone as a flashlight, you see big red lumps on both sides of your uvula (the hanging thing in the center). *Is this Strep?*

What's going on?

"Strep throat" is a bacterial infection caused by Group A Streptococcus.

Note that different Strep groups (B, C, D, and G) exist but typically cause other types of infections in the body. With a sore throat, however, doctors are primarily concerned about Group A Strep infections because this class of Strep has the unique potential to progress to more serious problems such as rheumatic fever (which can harm the heart valves), kidney damage, abscess formation near the tonsils, toxic shock, ear infections, and meningitis. **Diagnosing and treating Group A Strep infections in the throat prevents those serious complications.**

Treatment:

Good, old-fashioned **Penicillin** is the recommended treatment for Strep throat. In fact, if needles don't terrify you, one option is a single shot of penicillin (yes, in your gluteus, relatively high up—you only need to expose a few inches of skin). Oral penicillin tablets are given for ten days, and as always, it's important to take every pill. Do **not** stop taking the medication when your throat stops hurting, or you run the risk of developing the more serious complications of Strep. If you are truly allergic to penicillin, then obviously you will need a different antibiotic, and a single injection will not be an option for you.

Self-care includes over-the-counter pain and fever reducers ibuprofen (Advil) and acetaminophen (Tylenol); consider purchasing the liquid version in the children's section if swallowing pills is too painful.

Pain relieving throat sprays (like Chloraseptic or Cepacol) often end up numbing your lips and tongue more than your throat, so choose the liquid medications you can gargle, or perhaps a throat lozenge. Similarly, clinicians may prescribe lidocaine lollipops, which provide a stronger numbing medicine as you suck on them. However, in my clinical experience, only about half of patients like this product because, while this prescription anesthetic does indeed decrease the pain from your tonsils, it also numbs the majority of your tongue and mouth, giving some people the sensation of choking.

Gargling with warm salt water really does help with sore throats, including Strep throat. If you are going to use them, make sure the solution is very salty, because the point is to make the solution hypertonic (*check your chemistry text book if you're really curious*) so it pulls fluid out of the tissues, decreases swelling, and may also help with killing off the Strep bacteria. How much salt? No evidence-based studies give us a solid answer. My simple response is at least a teaspoon of salt in a cup of warm water, and honestly, I add more than that because the idea is to add more salt than will dissolve into the warm water when you stir it. *This mixture is not to drink—just gargle and spit out.*

Head to your doctor if:
- You've had mild–moderate symptoms for a few days and over-the-counter symptom treatment for a couple of days haven't helped.
- You felt totally fine then suddenly develop fever (temp greater than 100.4°F), a severe sore throat, and **no cough** or runny nose.
- You have a history of frequent Strep infections that were proven to be Strep by testing.
  - Documenting each infection helps your doctor decide when a tonsillectomy is appropriate; guidelines suggest removal if you have more than three Strep infections per year for three years, more than five per year for two years, or more than seven in one year.
  - Tonsillectomy may also be recommended for chronically enlarged tonsils that obstruct the airway while sleeping, causing snoring, interrupted sleep, and sleep apnea.

Worst-case scenario:

As noted above, untreated Strep can progress to very serious complications, including toxic shock, meningitis, and death. However, the worst-case scenario we typically see in the university setting is a **peritonsillar**

143

abscess, where a collection of bacteria and inflammation swells up enough to potentially block your airway.

What does a peritonsillar abscess look like? Upon examining the mouth, we see one side far more swollen than the other (not simply the tonsils, but the roof of the mouth near it), and the patient can often barely swallow their own saliva. All this swelling creates a "hot potato" voice—picture the muffled sound of your voice when you accidentally take a big bite of a burning-hot potato. Although some university health centers may be able to treat this situation, most of us will urgently transfer this patient to the care of an ENT (Ear, Nose, and Throat) surgeon for further treatment, which may be done either as an outpatient in the doctor's office or in a hospital.

Prevention:

Strep infections, like the common cold viruses, are spread via respiratory droplets. When someone with Strep coughs (which happily doesn't happen much) or sneezes, the bacteria are spread into the air on these droplets, which then land on something . . . like the handrail along stairs. The next person touches that rail with the bacteria, then uses their hand to rub their eyes, nose, or mouth, passing the bacteria into their own system. Of course, direct contact like kissing or sharing a fork or spoon will also easily pass the germs.

- **Hand washing**, therefore, is the best prevention to keep from getting Strep from strangers, and limiting intimate contact with anyone who is complaining of a fever or sore throat works with friends.
- **Sharing toothbrushes, drinks, or lip products will also spread germs**. In fact, if you have Strep, avoid reinfecting yourself by changing toothbrushes once you complete your antibiotics.

TIPS:
- If you have a cough with your sore throat, it's **not** Strep.
- If you have a runny nose and bad cough with your sore throat, it's **still not** Strep.

○ **Fever (temp higher than 100.5°F) + Painful, Swollen, Red Tonsils + Tender Swollen Front of the Neck Lymph Nodes + NO Cough = Strep**

○ **Rapid Strep tests** are wonderful when they are positive (less than 1 percent chance that they are inaccurate), but rapid Strep tests that are negative can be wrong up to 30 percent of the time (meaning they say you do not have Strep, but you do). This explains why we send a regular throat culture after a negative rapid test if we are pretty convinced you have Strep.

○ Even untreated sore throats caused by Strep will get less sore after several days, but *that does not decrease your chance of having complications from the Strep infection.*

○ All the above is true the vast majority of the time . . . but **yes, there are exceptions.** Some people with Strep have a slight cough, or never measured their temperature to know if they had a fever, or their tonsils are not the classic fire-engine bright red. However, these general rules should help you decide when it's more urgent to see your physician.

○ **Sometimes you have Strep,** *but you **also** have Infectious Mononucleosis.*

   ○ See Chapter 28: When Your Sore Throat Is Mono (page 146).

○ Sometimes you **think** you have Strep . . . *but it's a sexually transmitted infection.*

   ○ See Chapter 29: When Your Sore Throat Is . . . That Which Shall Not Be Named (page 149).

Chapter 28
When Your Sore Throat Is Mono

What If: My Sore Throat Is Mono?
Medical Name: Infectious Mononucleosis

What most likely happened:
Last week, you were diagnosed with Strep throat, and although you are halfway through your antibiotics and started to feel better a couple of days ago, now you've got a fever again, hugely swollen glands, nausea, and merely getting showered and heading to class seem impossible.

What's going on?
The Epstein-Barr Virus (EBV) causes mononucleosis (a.k.a. mono, or "the kissing disease"), an extremely common viral infection in college students. Yes, mono can be transmitted by kissing, but most people with mono catch it the same way you catch a cold—exposure to scattered respiratory droplets from an infected individual's cough or sneeze. Classic symptoms are high fevers, sore throat with inflamed, red tonsils, swollen glands (especially neck lymph nodes), fatigue, and possibly nausea or abdominal discomfort.

Treatment:

- **Rest, hydration,** and **time** are the primary treatments for mono, because we do not yet have any antiviral medications against this virus.
- **Antibiotics** should only be added if you also test positive for a secondary bacterial infection like Strep throat, which frequently piggybacks on mono.
- **Steroids** may be added to help shrink your tonsils if they become so enlarged that they could restrict or potentially close off your airway.

Head to your doctor if you have:

- Diagnosed Strep throat that isn't improving after several days of antibiotics.
- Unexplained fatigue or persistent nausea.
- Tender, swollen glands in your neck, armpits, or groin.

Worst-case scenario:

The vast majority of mono cases pretty much ground you for a week or two and then restrict any intensive activity for a couple months. However, some people get and stay sick enough that they need to drop a course or even take a medical leave for the semester.

Less than 1 percent of people with an acute mono infection will rupture their spleen, which is a life-threatening surgical emergency; this is why doctors advise **no sports activities** the first three to four weeks after diagnosis. *Percentage is low, but consequences are high*—**don't risk it!**

Prevention:

Same prevention as for the common cold:

- Frequent handwashing
- Not sharing drinks or utensils
- Optimizing your health with good nutrition and consistent sleep—exhausted bodies are more likely to catch viruses

TIPS:

○ By age thirty-five, 90 percent of people show blood test evidence that they have had mono, though **many** are unaware they did, because about 10 percent of mono infections have no symptoms, and another chunk of mono infections occur in childhood (when doctors choose not to draw blood to look for mono when little kids have high fevers and swollen glands). **Take-home message: if you get mono, *try not to overly stress about giving it to someone else*; many are already immune, and this disease is less contagious than the common cold.**

○ **The rapid "mono-spot" blood test is falsely negative 25 percent of the time the first week** of infection (meaning the test says you do **not** have mono, but you actually do). **Go back** and retest a week later if your symptoms are worse or not improving.

○ **Mono can enlarge your spleen,** so the first three weeks after mono diagnosis, we recommend **no** contact sports because an enlarged spleen can more easily rupture and cause serious internal bleeding.

○ **Not all mono shows up with high fevers and sore throat;** sometimes it's just nausea and fatigue, and rarely mono causes isolated nerve pain (an unexplained, sharp pain on one side of your face or body).

○ If you are diagnosed with mono, **tell your professors—*early communication is key if you may need extra time on a project, paper, or exam.***

○ If you are unfortunate enough to get a severe case of mono, ask your physician to direct you to your campus student disability services to discuss your options for a medically excused course load reduction or, if necessary, medical withdrawal for the semester.

Chapter 29

When Your Sore Throat Is . . . That Which Shall Not Be Named

What If: I Still Have a Sore Throat (But It's NOT Strep or Mono)?

Medical Name: Sexually Transmitted Infection (STI) Pharyngitis

What most likely happened:

You've got a nagging sore throat, and you can see white spots on your red, swollen tonsils. Your Strep test was negative last week, but since they told you to come back if you weren't better . . . here you are. Today's repeat rapid Strep test was negative, too, and since you had mono two years ago, that diagnosis is unlikely.

Could this be allergies? Doubtful without any sneezing, itchy eyes, or runny nose.

Another virus? Maybe, but most other viral infections don't cause swollen, patchy tonsils.

The doctor's next question throws you off guard:

"Any new sexual partners, including oral sex (meaning your mouth on your partner's genitals)?"

149

What? Your heart and brain race to the obvious conclusion, recalling a hookup two weekends ago . . .

What's going on?

The United States reports over two million annual cases of chlamydia and gonorrhea, with nearly half occurring in young people ages fifteen to twenty-four. *We treat these **all the time** on college campuses.* While the majority of these STIs are located in the genital area, we also see them in the mouth. However, the truth is that many oral/throat STIs have minimal symptoms (so people ignore them and don't seek treatment), and, frankly, many clinicians don't think about nongenital STIs (translation: tests never ordered). Fortunately, medical education and standardized guidelines for testing "extragenital" sites (throat and rectum) are rapidly evolving, as are the tests themselves.

The myth persists that oral sex is "safe," despite the fact that nearly all STIs are easily transmitted through oral-genital intimacy. Although an estimated half of college students engage in oral sex, only a fraction of them consistently use condoms/barriers with this activity. Gonorrhea is the most common bacterial culprit for oral STIs, twice as common in men who have sex with men (MSM), but certainly also seen in men who have sex with women (MSW).

Treatment:

- Antibiotics, typically more than one. Gonorrhea travels so frequently with chlamydia that current guidelines dictate automatic treatment for both if you test positive for gonorrhea, which means you will get a shot (in the hip) of the antibiotic ceftriaxone, plus a single large dose of the oral antibiotic azithromycin.
- Every STI treatment should include testing for other STIs. Why? Because it's the same mode of transmission, so if you've got one, you easily may have another (and many are silent).
  - See Chapter 45: Sexually Transmitted Infections (Yes, It Happens to People like You) on page 221.

Head to your doctor if:

- You develop a sore throat or painful swallowing, especially within one to three weeks after giving unprotected (no barrier) oral sex.
- You've been sexually active and would like STI testing (blood for HIV, Hep C, and syphilis; urine test plus oral and rectal swabs for gonorrhea and chlamydia).

Worst-case scenario:

- The most concerning thing about gonorrheal infections is that most of our antibiotics no longer work against these bacteria. We are down to one effective class of antibiotic that works, so the worst case is contracting a strain of gonorrhea that is resistant to this treatment.
- Untreated oral gonorrhea may have minimal symptoms yet can still be spread from your mouth to your partner's genitals through unprotected (no barrier used) oral sex, so the other worst case is not realizing you have this infection and passing it on to a new partner.
- Untreated gonorrhea that spreads throughout your body can cause multiple complications within your joints, eyes, and reproductive system, including a risk of infertility.

Prevention:

- If you are sexually active, use a barrier between your mouth and your partner's genitals for oral sex (condom for male recipients; dental dam for female recipients).
- *Blood and urine STI testing do not detect oral or anal gonorrheal/chlamydia infections*; a throat or anal swab must be used. Be sure you are tested for STIs at all sites where you have intimate sexual contact.

TIPS:

- ○ Oral sex is the only reason *flavored condoms* were invented . . . if you choose this type of intimacy, use them!
- ○ *Almost every sexually transmitted infection can be passed via oral sex,* but consistently using a barrier dramatically decreases this risk.
- ○ Although condoms do rarely break (between 2 to 10 percent of usage), *far more condom "failures" are from not actually using condoms* (because you forgot, were drunk, embarrassed to ask, etc.). Again, use them!

Chapter 30
College Is a
Pain in the Neck

What If: My Neck Hurts?
Medical Name: Cervical Strain

What most likely happened:

Necks are not designed for extended forced flexion, which is exactly what happens with cell phones and laptops. Studies show that more than half of college students are addicted to their cell phones, spending up to ten hours per day glued to the screen. Campuses are filled with universally bent heads and hunched shoulders, texting

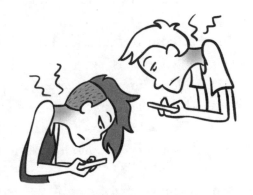

away while walking, sitting, eating . . . and scarily while biking or driving. Now add in laptops, which, by themselves, cannot be ergonomically correct, because if your arms are relaxed by your side and your elbows bent to roughly 90 degrees, your head and shoulders will have to be flexed and bent or hunched to see the screen. Not surprisingly, stiff, painful necks are a common complaint.

What's going on?

A flexed neck increases the forces on your spine, effectively increasing the weight of your head from roughly ten pounds at a neutral position to nearly sixty pounds when flexed sixty degrees. Constant flexion weakens your neck and back (especially trapezius and rhomboid) muscles, worsening your head-forward posture, which further strains your muscles and creates a negative loop. Don't wait until your dull-aching, stiff neck goes into intense spasm and pain to seek help.

Treatment:

- Starts with OTC pain relievers acetaminophen (Tylenol) and ibuprofen (Advil/Motrin).
- Topical cool or heat packs.
- Ergonomic assessment (and implementation of corrective changes) for phone, desktop, and, most important, your laptop.
- Stretching and strengthening exercises (with formal physical therapy instruction if available).

Head to your doctor if your:

- Neck pain is severe.
- Neck pain persists despite OTC pain relievers, stretching, and behavior modification.
- Pain radiates down your shoulder/arm or up to your head.
- Arms are weak, numb, or tingling.

Worst-case scenario:

Untreated neck pain can progress to chronic neck pain and degenerative (arthritic) problems.

Prevention:

- Purchase a laptop desk if you work on your bed.

- If you primarily use a laptop, get a portable keyboard so you can position your laptop to line up your eyes level with the screen and put your keyboard lower so your arms are relaxed at your side and elbows bent comfortably around 90 degrees.
- While on your laptop, set an alarm for at least every hour and take thirty to sixty seconds to stand up and gently stretch your neck left (hold for ten seconds) and right, then put your arms/shoulders through a gentle range of motion stretches, too.
- Consider a weekly yoga or core-strengthening class.

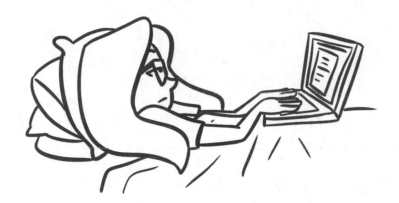

TIPS:

- ○ Avoid lying flat on your back with your head propped with pillows or the headboard.
- ○ Texting or browsing your social media? Raise the phone up to your eye level, rather than bending your head forward.
- ○ **Neck pain often responds well to massage**; this is the perfect excuse to check out any discounted massage services your university may offer.
  - ○ Many campus rec centers now offer massage therapy services as well as personal training at their gyms—I highly recommend both!

Chapter 31
Something's Stuck in My Throat

What If: Something Gets Stuck in My Throat?
Medical Name: Esophageal Abrasion/Spasm

What most likely happened:
Scenario A: "Last night, I had a bad headache, so I took two ibuprofen tablets right before I went to bed, "dry-swallowing" them without any water or other liquid. I woke up this morning, and I'm pretty sure one got stuck in my throat! It hurts a ton in one specific spot."

Scenario B: "I was eating chips and queso at a Mexican restaurant, and suddenly one got stuck in my throat, and I can't make it go down. That happened at lunch yesterday, and it still feels stuck, even though I've eaten other food and drunk a ton of water."

Scenario C: Tailgate party, eating hotdogs or burgers with friends, talking and laughing, and suddenly you are choking and coughing because the meat went "down the wrong pipe," and you are unable to breathe.

What's going on?
In scenarios A and B, something DOES get temporarily stuck or at least scrapes the inside lining of your esophagus. There is no trouble breathing,

no forced coughing or choking, because this problem is in the food pipe (esophagus), not the air pipe (trachea). Although it definitely **feels** like the pill or chip is still sitting there in your throat, the vast majority of the time, what you are dealing with is a leftover irritation—a superficial scrape that hurts like crazy, but no object remains physically stuck in your throat.

In scenario C, food did not go down the esophagus but actually went into your airway. Obviously, this is a medical emergency, and the first step is performing the Heimlich maneuver (if your own forceful coughing doesn't send the food flying out of your mouth).

Treatment:

When the lining of the esophagus is irritated for any reason, treatment focuses on interventions to reduce further injury from both above (more food or pills coming down) and below (stomach acid refluxing back up).

- **Dietary changes:**
  - Eat a mechanically soft diet for a few days
    - yogurt, mashed potatoes, applesauce, soup
- **Stop Alcohol, Nicotine, Caffeine, and Peppermint**
  - These substances all cause acid reflux, meaning that they allow more stomach acid to flow back up into the esophagus. Curious how? Just above the stomach is a band of tissue (the lower esophageal sphincter) that opens to allow food to enter the stomach but then closes to keep the acid confined to the stomach, protecting the more fragile lining of the esophagus. These substances all relax that sphincter, allowing it to open and thus splash some food and acid back upstream. Think about what people traditionally have done after eating too much at a restaurant: they order coffee, an after-dinner alcoholic beverage, smoke a cigarette, or grab a mint on the way out. Why? Because all these substances work to open that sphincter, effectively expanding the volume for your overly "stuffed stomach" and thereby making you feel less full.

- **Medications to decrease stomach acid**
  - Antacids (neutralize the acid directly):
    - Calcium carbonate (Tums)
    - Aluminum hydroxide (Mylanta)
    - Aluminum/ magnesium/simethicone (Maalox)
  - H-2 Blockers (decrease acid production):
    - Cimetidine (Tagamet)
    - Famotidine (Pepcid/Zantac 360)
    - Nizatidine (Axid)
  - Proton Pump Inhibitors (decrease acid production even more)
    - Omeprazole (Prilosec)
    - Esomeprazole (Nexium)
    - Lansoprazole (Prevacid)
    - Rabeprazole (Aciphex)
    - Pantoprazole (Protonix)
- **Medication that forms a barrier, coating the injured areas**
  - Sucralfate (Carafate)
- **Endoscopy**
  - Performed by a Gastroenterologist (GI doctor)—a scope directly visualizes your esophagus to definitively diagnosis and potentially treat via dilation if there is any obstructive narrowing present.

When to head to your doctor:
- **Intense pain: do *not* wait,** head to your doctor.
- **Mild to Moderate pain**: consider trying dietary changes and OTC medications listed above for a day; see the doctor if any worsening or not steadily improving.
- Any problems breathing, seek emergent care (you're in college, you know this).

Worst-case scenario:

A "stuck" pill can chemically eat into the lining of your esophagus, creating an ulcer (picture a scrape that can ooze and bleed) or even an actual hole that would need to be surgically corrected. These ulcers can lead to scarring that partially closes or obstructs the esophagus, causing painful and ineffective swallowing.

Young people in their teens or twenties rarely get an actual piece of food stuck in their throats, though this is not infrequently seen in an older population. The most common perpetrator is an overly large bite of steak. If this chunk of food becomes truly stuck, the worst case is surgical removal via an endoscopic procedure (instruments maneuvered down your throat while you are sedated).

Food, pills, or other objects stuck in the trachea create **airway** emergencies. The worst-case scenario is literally death by choking. Fortunately, these life-threatening situations are not common in the college-aged crowd.

Prevention:

- **Never ever** "dry-swallow pills."
- Take **one** pill at a time. (*Stop popping in three ibuprofens or vitamins at once!*)
- **Drink** a couple of ounces (at least **half a glass**) of water or other liquid with every single pill you swallow.
- Wait at least ten minutes before lying down after taking pills (let gravity do its thing).
- Cut up your food into smaller bites than you think is necessary and **chew well**.

TIPS:

- o If you feel like a piece of food is stuck in your throat, and your breathing is **not** affected at all (so you know it's your esophagus, not your trachea), consider trying to drink a few ounces of Coke. Though the mechanism is not understood, a few small studies in the early 1990s showed this may be helpful.

○ Start OTC meds with a **liquid antacid** such as brand or generic Maalox or Mylanta; although it doesn't actually "coat" like the prescription sucralfate, they often provide an appreciable degree of immediate relief.

○ Check labels to **choose smaller-sized, coated tablets** when possible (especially pain relievers and vitamins).

○ When swallowing pills, place the medication in your mouth, take a sip of water, then tilt your chin toward your chest for capsules or lift your back slightly for tablets **before** you actually swallow. Why? Because capsules float, so leaning forward actually moves them to the back of your throat, making it easier to swallow.

○ **Don't be embarrassed if you have trouble swallowing pills—** you are not the only one in college who "never learned how," so please tell your doctor! Odds are good you have a strong gag reflex that makes it extra challenging for you. What else can you do?

　○ Talk with your doctor to see if there is a liquid alternative.

　○ Talk with your pharmacist and ask if your prescription can be crushed (most pills can, but anything coated or time-released usually cannot). If so, crush the pill with the back of a spoon and mix it into a spoonful of pudding or applesauce (two foods that are easily stored in dorms because they don't require refrigeration and they come in single-serving packages).

　○ Practice swallowing pills with mini M&Ms placed on the front of your tongue, using a big glass of water. *People often suggest putting the pill "way back" . . . and that just gags you.*

Chapter 32
My Heart Is Fluttering–
Palpitations and Panic

What If: My Heart Is Skipping, Flip-Flopping, or Racing?

Medical Name: Palpitations and Panic Attacks

What most likely happened:

It's been happening off and on for weeks, but last night, when you were desperately trying to fall asleep, your heart kept flip-flopping and randomly stuttering . . . making you anxious, which sped up your heart rate and worsened the skipping beats. Today, you can't shake the feeling that there is something seriously wrong with your heart, although other than racing a bit, it seems to be beating normally.

What's going on?

Otherwise healthy college students commonly end up with palpitations from something (or a combination of things) they put in their mouths:

- **Drinks:** caffeine and alcohol
- **Smoking:** nicotine and marijuana
- **OTC meds:** decongestants (pseudoephedrine) and antihistamines

- **Prescription meds**: Asthma inhalers, ADHD (Attention Deficit Hyperactivity Disorder)
- **OTC supplements**: workout or energy boosters and diet pills

All these substances can speed up your heart rate or trigger early, extra beats (which is the "flop" that you feel). Typically, we see students who use one of these items regularly (like caffeine) but then get a cold and add in a decongestant/antihistamine combination, or start taking ADHD meds, or start vaping or binge-drinking, and *it's the second or third added-on substance that pushes their heart irritability over the threshold.*

Stress: College life overflows with potential stressors, from academic challenges, finances, and career choices to every type of relationship roller coaster. Not surprisingly, anxiety is another common cause of palpitations. The adrenaline from anxiety speeds up your heart dramatically, causing that racing/fluttering sensation. If you escalate to a panic attack, you may also experience chest tightness, shortness of breath, hot flashes or chills, nausea, trembling, a sense of impending doom, and often numbness or tingling around your mouth, fingers, and toes (from hyperventilating). The worst part about panic attacks is that, frequently, there is not an identifiable trigger, which leaves you fearful of exactly when and where the next one might occur. The good news is that panic attacks and the vast majority of palpitations are not inherently dangerous, though they can be very upsetting to experience.

Less common medical causes:

- Anemia (do you have heavy periods, or have you been vegetarian for a long time?)
- Heart valve issues, like mitral valve prolapse
- Supraventricular Tachycardias (SVT)
- Hyperthyroidism
- Atrial fibrillation/flutter (rare in teens/early twenties)
- Abnormal electrolytes

Treatment:

Assuming your medical workup ruled out other medical causes, the treatment will focus on stopping the substances triggering or aggravating your symptoms.

- Switching from an oral decongestant to nasal steroid sprays
- Adding oral asthma medications (like Singulair) or increasing steroid inhalers to decrease need for short-acting inhalers (which cause the racing heart)
- Changing ADHD medications to a less or nonstimulating drug
- Weaning down (and off) caffeine, alcohol, nicotine, and pot

Direct treatment to minimize palpitations is typically a daily prescription medication that slows down your heart rate such as metoprolol (Toprol XL or Lopressor). This drug is very commonly prescribed for stage fright and other social phobias.

Anxiety treatment starts with specific counseling called **cognitive behavioral therapy (CBT).**

- CBT "talk therapy" helps people recognize how they are unconsciously magnifying and catastrophizing potential negative outcomes, which then triggers the physical anxiety responses like shortness of breath, a racing or flip-flopping heart, tremors, etc.

Depending on the severity and frequency of your symptoms, daily preventative medications may be added:

- Selective Serotonin Reuptake Inhibitors (SSRIs) such as fluoxetine (Prozac), paroxetine (Paxil), or sertraline (Zoloft)
- Serotonin and norepinephrine reuptake inhibitors (SNRIs) like venlafaxine (Effexor)

Head to your doctor if you have:

- New palpitations or a racing heart without explanation.

- Palpitations (with or without an explanation) that are distracting or upsetting you.
- Shortness of breath or decreased exercise tolerance.
- Nearly or actually passed out.

Worst-case scenario:

Palpitations and racing heartbeats are infrequently the result of a genetic heart conduction issue or another dangerously fast or irregular heart rhythm. These uncommon problems may be detected with a standard EKG, but they will require additional specialist testing and treatment.

Prevention:

- Recognize the possible triggers and cut back on everything optional.
- Don't smoke (anything).
- Maximize your health: good nutrition, daily exercise, and consistent sleep patterns.

TIPS:

- **Workout and weight loss supplements are notorious** for causing palpitations, primarily because of high concentrations of caffeine. *Avoid them!*
- **Consistent daily aerobic exercise** (enough to raise your heart rate for approximately thirty minutes—doesn't have to be fancier than walking) **can improve anxiety and depression** as much as a low dose of an antidepressant/antianxiety medication.
- **The Valsalva maneuver** (either holding your nose and blowing against resistance or "bearing down" in your abdomen) can often stimulate your vagal nerve enough to **slow down** a rapid heart rate.

Chapter 33

I Can't Stop Coughing–
Is This Bronchitis?
Flu? Pneumonia?

What If: I Can't Stop Coughing?

Medical Names: Bronchitis, Pneumonia, Upper Respiratory Infection, Lower Respiratory Infection, Postviral Cough, or Reactive Airways

What most likely happened:

Some point in the last week or two, you had a few days of fever, sore throat, stuffy nose and perhaps some body aches. After testing negative for COVID and the flu, you were reassured that it was "just a common cold." However, this darn cough is still hanging on and driving you nuts. And . . . driving your classmates and roommate nuts, too. You've gone through a bottle of cough syrup and several bags of cough drops, and when you complain, everyone says "go see a doctor to get some antibiotics" to make your cough go away.

What's going on?

After a viral respiratory infection, the inflammatory defense system in your lungs may become overly reactive, creating too much mucus, which then triggers subsequent spasm of the airways, producing persistent coughing and wheezing. Though asthma has different triggers (allergens, cold air, other environmental triggers), this process is virtually the same, and therefore, treatment may involve asthma medications.

Are you still infected? **Probably not.** The prolonged cough after respiratory infections can last up to **six weeks**, which is why **cough** earns gold, silver, or bronze virtually every year for the top reasons people see their primary care doctors.

Is this bronchitis? Very possibly, because **acute bronchitis is defined as inflammation of the large airways (including the trachea)** *without evidence of pneumonia.* Bronchitis is a "clinical diagnosis," which means that your doctor decides this from your exam, rather than a specific test like a rapid Strep test. What would be "evidence of pneumonia"? Although not always clinically obvious, pneumonia infections typically create fast breathing, rapid heart rates, fevers, and specific sounds heard with a stethoscope over the affected area. If these physical signs do not accompany your ugly cough, your diagnosis will likely be "bronchitis," although "viral bronchitis" or "chest cold" might be a better label to emphasize that antibiotics are not the answer.

How can you tell if you need antibiotics?

Here we have the art as much as the science of medicine. Frankly, without the benefit of a stethoscope, otoscope, thermometer, pulse oximeter (to measure oxygen level), possibly blood tests, and, rarely, X-rays, none of us can "just tell" which patients definitively need antibiotics. As noted above, the presence of pneumonia signs and symptoms helps your doctor decide which further testing is necessary, if any.

Please note that **green mucus does not equal bacterial infection.** Green, brown, yellow, and even blood-streaked mucus can occur with progressive inflammation and irritation in the mucus membranes that line your nose and respiratory tract, whether your infection is viral or bacterial. Chronic allergic inflammation plus overdrying antihistamines are a common culprit of brown or blood-stained mucus, especially upon blowing your nose first thing in the morning. Additionally, the reverse is true: you can have beautifully clear mucus but still have a bacterial infection (though admittedly less common). Therefore, it's less about the color of your snot and more about the story.

You may need antibiotics IF you have several days to a week of stuffy nose, aches, cough, etc., that are starting to slowly improve, and then *boom*—you are hit with a second round of fever, chills, and sudden worsening of symptoms. *Why does this happen?* The initial viral infection broke down your intact nasal membranes and respiratory tract, linings that are the body's first line of defense, so now bacteria can more easily enter your system and set up shop.

Treatment:

OTC cough medications:
- DM (dextromethorphan: example, Delsym): works at the brain level, decreasing the drive to cough
- Guaifenesin (example, Mucinex) thins up the mucus, so easier to cough up—hence, "expectorant"
- Combinations of these ingredients (along with decongestants to help stuffy noses) make up the cough/cold/flu products like Dayquil/Nyquil/Robitussin, etc., and may be helpful in alleviating cough and cold symptoms in adults.

Menthol: Old-fashioned vapor rubs and menthol-containing cough drops may indeed help with coughs.

- **Fun fact:** Menthol cigarettes were created because menthol is a mild anesthetic (numbs the throat to tolerate inhaling hot vapor) and also suppresses the cough reflex.

Nonmedicinal treatments:
- **Humidifiers** add moisture to the air and can ease coughs (remember that the overdrying antihistamines can make mucus dry and sticky, tougher to cough up and out, thus aggravating coughs).

- **Cool mist versus warm vaporizer?** No difference in your body (the moist air is the same temperature by the time it hits your lungs), but the heated vaporizer adds the risk of an accidental burn, especially in tight quarters like dorm rooms, so cool mist humidifiers are preferable.
- For any machine, empty remaining water, replacing it with fresh water daily, and **clean** your device (empty the water, dry all surfaces, and clean with bleach wipes or a diluted bleach solution) every two to three days.
- **Honey*** has been objectively shown to help improve coughs; try a teaspoonful straight up or added to a cup of hot tea. (*Never for kids younger than one year old.)

Prescription medications:
- **"Asthma" inhalers:**
  - **Albuterol inhaler:** Directly pops open the small airways in your lungs
  - **Steroid inhaler or steroid pills:** Suppress the inflammatory response responsible for the cough-triggering excess mucus production and subsequent airway spasm
- **Benzonatate (trade name Tessalon):** Nonaddictive, nonsedating medication that works in the lungs to decrease the cough reflex by numbing the stretch receptors in the respiratory tract
- **Codeine or hydrocodone cough syrups:** *Addictive*, works at the brain level to suppress cough.
  - **Please** do not walk into your doctor asking for these addictive narcotic medications. A short-term prescription may be indicated for a cough that is keeping you (and your roommates) awake all night, especially if you are already taking other OTC and prescription cough suppressants. However, many physicians have stopped prescribing this class of drugs altogether in an effort to help end the opioid crisis in the United States.

- Additionally, in a college population where binge-drinking is common, conscientious doctors are nervous about the potential intentional or unintentional mixing of these sedating drugs with alcohol. Combined, narcotics plus alcohol **suppress your drive to breathe** and put you at high risk of accidental death. Therefore, if you **do** get a prescription for a narcotic cough syrup, please keep it in a locked drawer and *never* mix with alcohol.
- **Antibiotics:** Infrequently needed, but they are required for bacterial pneumonias, including the typically less severe "walking pneumonia," which is caused by Mycoplasma bacteria. Note that current standard of care is to avoid antibiotics for "bronchitis," now recognized to be viral the vast majority of the time.

Head to your doctor if:
- Your cough was improving, but suddenly you get worse with fever, chills, shortness of breath, fits of coughing, or coughing that is waking you up (or keeping you up)—it's time to be examined.
- Your cough lasts longer than three weeks (and/or is not steadily improving).
- You can't sleep because of the cough.
- You have asthma, or if you feel chest pressure, tightness, or shortness of breath.
- You see blood in your mucus—don't freak out, this is not uncommon—but it's time to be examined.
- You feel progressively weaker and out of energy.

Worst-case scenario:
Infectious coughs can progress to pneumonia, which ranges from easily managed bacterial walking pneumonia to potentially lethal viral pneumonias. Every year, otherwise healthy people die from the flu this way, which is exactly why doctors are so hot on flu vaccines. The same can be said for COVID-19.

Prevention:

- **Hand Washing:** Nothing beats consistent, thorough hand washing to prevent the spread of germs. *Don't splash and dash—* remember to cleanse for at least twenty seconds to be fully effective, whether using soap and water or sanitizer.
- **Flu Vaccine:** Especially during college, where you share space with literally thousands of other people, take advantage of your school's free or very inexpensive flu shot clinics every September. ***Flu shots aren't perfect, but they definitely decrease the severity of the flu if you become infected.***
- **COVID-19 Vaccine:** Similarly, the COVID vaccines are the best defense against severe disease, hospitalization, and death from COVID.

TIPS:

- **Avoid touching things** people routinely touch, like escalator or stair **handrails** and, when possible, doorknobs (look for automatic press pads you can bump with your arm or hip).
- If you are experiencing FITS of coughing so hard that it makes you gag and even vomit, go to the doctor—this may be Whooping Cough, which is a bacterial infection (caused by Bordetella pertussis) and, therefore, can be treated with antibiotics.
- Did I mention annual **Flu Vaccines**?
    - If you're terrified of needles, most years you should be able to receive the nasal spray vaccine (unless you have asthma).
    - *The flu vaccine does NOT cause the flu.*
    - **The flu vaccine doesn't make you bulletproof for all infections** (meaning you can still catch colds and stomach viruses).
    - **As a healthy, young college student, are you likely to die from the flu?** No, though sadly, the flu does kill some otherwise healthy young people every year. Vaccine expert

Gretchen LaSalle, MD, reminds us that "looking back at those people who died from the flu, we see that 80 to 90 percent of them did not get the flu shot that year. Don't let perfect be the enemy of good. If you're waiting for the perfect vaccine, you're going to die waiting . . . possibly of a vaccine-preventable disease." The bigger concern is that **real flu** knocks you off your feet for a full week with terrible headaches, fever, sore throat, cough, chills, nausea, and muscle aches like a Mack truck mowed you down . . . not exactly ideal when you need to be in class, doing projects, or studying for exams. What we see in our campus clinic every year is that the vaccinated students who still end up with the flu have a far milder case of the flu, missing only a day or two of classes, versus the unimmunized students with the flu who miss a week or more.

Chapter 34
I Can't Catch My Breath (Common): Asthma

What If: I Start Wheezing?

Medical Name: Asthma or Reactive Airways Disease

What most likely happened:

Scenario A: As a child, you were diagnosed with asthma and had to use inhalers, but you haven't used one since before high school. Now what started as stuffy nose cold symptoms has become a bad cough that makes your chest feel tight and leaves you short of breath.

Scenario B: You've committed to running a 10K with your roommate next month, but you can't seem to run more than about half a mile because, fairly consistently, about five to ten minutes after starting, your chest tightens up, you start coughing, and you have to stop completely to catch your breath. You can last longer on a treadmill in the gym, but you'd rather be outside in the brisk November air so you don't sweat so much.

Scenario C: Your new roommate is a smoker (only smokes out on the deck), and his German shepherd "Moose" is awesome, but dog hair blankets your apartment. Your frat has you spending way too many hours building and painting a massive stage and backdrop for the biggest party of the semester, and now you've got an annoying cough that's getting progressively worse.

What's going on?

Asthma is basically overreactive airways that secrete too much mucus and spasm shut in response to a variety of triggers:

- allergens (pollen, molds, etc.)
- smoking/vaping
- respiratory infections
- cold air
- exercise

Treatment:

- **Albuterol or Levalbuterol Inhalers** (Proventil, Ventolin, Proair, Xopenex, etc.)
  - These "rescue" inhalers immediately pop open small airways to transiently increase air flow and ease symptoms; effects are not long-lasting.
  - Help you feel better in the short term but don't fix the inflammation problem causing those symptoms.
  - May be used preventatively right before activity for exercise-induced asthma.
  - May be used as needed for immediate relief of symptoms.
  - Major side effect is racing heart and hand tremors (make you feel like you've had too much caffeine).
- **Steroid Inhalers** (Flovent, Pulmicort, Asmanex, Qvar, etc.)
  - Kick in slowly but critical for treatment because they fix the root problem, inflammation, and airway swelling.
- **Oral Steroids** (Prednisone)
  - Often prescribed short term for acute asthma exacerbations
- **Nebulizer**
  - Machine used in clinics and ERs (and occasionally prescribed for home use) when puffs from an inhaler aren't enough to relieve asthma symptoms

- "Neb" breathing treatments deliver the rapid-acting albuterol solutions (plus/minus a steroid or other medication) in a continuous mist through a mouthpiece or mask.
- **Combination Inhalers**
  - Steroid plus a long-acting version of the albuterol-type airway opener
  - More convenient, but more expensive
  - Equally effective as using separate inhalers of the same medications
- **Additional Medications Used Less Commonly:**
  - Leukotriene modifiers (Singulair, Zyflo, Accolate)
    - Daily oral medication that decreases the inflammatory process, similar to steroids but with different side effects
  - Ipratropium (Atrovent)
    - Short-acting inhaler that helps relax airway muscles and dries secretions to increase air flow
  - Theophylline
    - Older asthma medication with multiple side effects, infrequently used
  - Biologics (omalizumab, mepolizumab, etc.)
    - New class of medications given as a shot or IV infusion every 2 to 8 weeks for moderate-to-severe asthma not controlled with other medications

Head to your doctor if you:
- Experience chest tightness, cough, or shortness of breath routinely during exercise, especially in cold weather.
- Have a worsening cough or wheezing during or after a respiratory infection.
- Are diagnosed with asthma and have to use your inhalers more than prescribed.

Worst-case scenario:

A severe, potentially life-threatening asthma exacerbation can happen to anyone with asthma, even if your symptoms are infrequent or mild; *do NOT underestimate your need for medical help*. **Asthma is a medical emergency if:**

- **You've used your rescue inhaler and your shortness of breath doesn't improve.**
- **Your chest muscles are straining to breathe.**
- **Your heart is racing (more than 120 beats per minute).**
- **You're struggling to talk because of lack of air.**

Severe exacerbations literally shut down your breathing; and, worst case, if breathing treatments and IV medications fail, you could be placed on artificial ventilation life support.

Prevention:

- Don't smoke. **Anything**. Yes, that includes vaping.
- If you are nineteen or older, get a pneumonia vaccine (Pneumovax 23: one-time shot for all adults diagnosed with asthma).
- Get your annual flu vaccine early; most colleges offer free or low-cost shot clinics in September.
- Immunotherapy with allergy shots (if you have identified specific allergies unresponsive to other medications)

TIPS:

- ○ *Stop inhaling anything besides air!* Specifically, stop using tobacco, e-cigs, and pot. *Seriously!* We can give you all the inhalers in the world, but if you keep irritating your lungs, our medications will not be enough.
- ○ Skip personal perfume or cologne.
- ○ Talk to your doctor about projects, jobs, or environments that might affect your asthma.

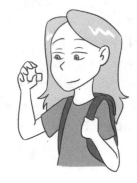

- Limit time working in chemistry labs (not so much the once-per-week class; more a weekly job setting up the chemicals).
- Limit frat/sorority pledge painting projects with prolonged exposure to paint fumes and solvents.
- Limit working with animals (pet dander).
- Limit working with small children (exposure to their many respiratory viruses).

- Using a **spacer** with your inhaler greatly increases the amount that reaches your lungs (rather than coating your mouth); an **empty toilet paper roll** works well if you don't have a manufactured one.
- Be sure to rinse out your mouth with water after using a steroid inhaler (to avoid getting thrush, a fungal mouth infection).
- Keep an extra albuterol (rapid-acting) inhaler in your backpack so you always have one.

Chapter 35

I Can't Catch My Breath + Chest Pain (Uncommon): Partially Collapsed Lung

What If: I Have Chest Pain? (Uncommon Cause: Collapsed Lung)

Medical Name: Primary Spontaneous Pneumothorax

What most likely happened:

You're the basketball prototype—lanky, tall, and thin—and although you haven't been sick or worked out too hard, you suddenly have an intense or nagging one-sided chest or back pain and some shortness of breath, with or without coughing, fatigue, and a racing heart. Changing positions doesn't help, and any type of exertion seems to make you work to catch your breath.

Or same body type, but you simply have unexplained sudden chest or back discomfort that won't go away (but no cough, racing heart, or obvious shortness of breath).

Or you were in a car accident last weekend, and the pain in your chest is getting worse instead of better.

What's going on?

In our typically healthy college population, most students are blissfully unaware that sudden chest pain could be a sign of a partially collapsed lung (pneumothorax—literally "air" in the chest). In fact, odds are they've never heard of lungs spontaneously deflating. Though not terribly common, spontaneous lung collapse occurs frequently enough (roughly twelve cases per 100,000 men and three per 100,000 women) that large college communities treat several every semester.

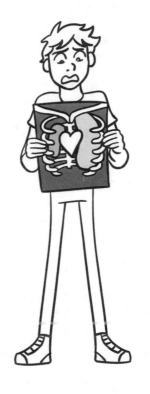

Though clearly not "spontaneous," lungs can also collapse as a result of trauma. No one would ignore a knife or gunshot wound, but blunt chest trauma like car accidents (with or without airbags) can also collapse a lung, and symptoms may be written off to expected muscle soreness.

Inflated lungs look like a swollen, soaked sponge, completely filling the chest cavity and leaving virtually no space between the lung tissue and the chest wall. However, if there is a rupture that allows air to leak into this potential space, the trapped air creates pressure that steadily compresses the lung, pushing downward and preventing the lung from fully inflating. Small air leaks typically have mild symptoms, so people may not seek care for several days. If, however, the air leak is large, this pressure can potentially collapse that lung into a shrunken lump unable to function, leaving its owner with chest tightness, pain, coughing, and intense difficulty breathing.

Treatment:

The good news is that simple observation is the treatment of choice for a first-time, small pneumothorax. We occasionally give supplemental oxygen, watch your symptoms, listen to your lungs, and look at serial X-rays over several days to weeks, ensuring your lung is slowly filling back up all the way. The bad news is that larger pockets of air (and therefore more compressed lungs) need to have that air removed so the lung can reinflate, which must be done in a hospital setting using a thin needle or a larger surgical chest tube. The worst news is that if you have this happen more than once, you may end up needing chest surgery to permanently fix the problem.

Head to your doctor if:
- You develop sudden, unexplained chest (or back) pain and shortness of breath.
- You have chest pain after scuba diving or high-altitude climbing.
- You develop chest pain or shortness of breath after any type of intense collision involving your chest (sports, scooters, bikes, or cars).

Worst-case scenario:

A partially collapsed lung can progress to a fully collapsed lung, which is (duh) a medical emergency that can be fatal without intervention. This is not usually subtle; don't worry you will miss the signs: greatly intensified pain, shortness of breath, racing heart, anxiety, and possibly passing out. (ER television dramas love to portray this with the doctors yelling they need to insert a chest tube, and indeed, that is the answer.)

Prevention:

- **Do not smoke *anything*!** *All types of inhaled smoke damage your lung tissue.*
- Both **high-altitude hiking** and **scuba diving** can create pressurized air leaks that create a pneumothorax. Therefore, strictly follow the safety guidelines both descending and ascending to avoid rapid changes in air pressure.
- **Wear seat belts** and avoid high-impact injuries.

TIPS:

- O A partially collapsed lung is not always dramatic, *so don't blow off persistent unexplained chest pain*, especially if you have any of these risk factors, such as if you:
  - O Are a tall, thin male
  - O Smoke
  - O Play football, hockey, or any other heavy contact sport
  - O Did extreme high-altitude climbing or scuba diving before your chest pain started

Chapter 36

Birth Control Pills + Chest Pain = Serious Problem (Till Proven Otherwise)

What If: Your Chest Pain Is from an Uncommon Cause (Blood Clot in Your Lung)?

Medical Name: Pulmonary Embolism

What most likely happened:

You are a female college student on birth control pills, and last weekend you survived an eight-hour-long, miserable middle-seat-squeezed-between-two-sleeping-humans flight back from studying abroad. Now your chest feels tight, your heart won't stop racing, and as you walk to class, you start coughing and can't seem to catch your breath. Your legs may seem completely normal, or one of your calves may appear swollen, tender, or red.

NOTE: If you are a female college student who takes birth control pills (*or a transgender person taking female hormone therapy*), and you call your campus clinic saying you are having ANY type of chest pain or shortness of breath, *you will likely be asked to come straight in to be examined.* While your chest pain or shortness of breath is far more likely to be coming from your chest muscles, GI tract (heartburn), or asthma, our job is to be sure you are not having the serious, much less common problem of a blood clot in your lungs. These clots can form in the lungs but more typically they quietly form in the calves and travel to the lungs.

What's going on?

Several common risk factors increase your chance of forming leg clots (deep vein thromboses) that can then migrate to the lungs to wreak havoc (pulmonary emboli):

- Estrogen (manufactured in your body or taken as a prescription medicine)
- Prolonged sitting
    - Primarily trips of more than four hours where you cannot get up and move around, like a cramped plane flight; however, around midterms or finals, we see this from sitting in front of a computer or at a desk studying all day
- Smoking
- Recent surgery
- Pregnancy
- Being overweight

College students frequently combine many of these risk factors, especially smoking, birth control use, and prolonged sitting.

How common are blood clots? And are they only from "the Pill"?

Let's get perspective from these annual estimates:

How many women are likely to get a blood clot based on their hormonal status?

- One to five women out of 10,000 healthy, nonpregnant women
- **Three to nine women out of 10,000** healthy, nonpregnant women taking oral contraceptive pills
    - **Roughly threefold increased risk by taking "the pill"**

- Five to twenty women out of 10,000 healthy **pregnant** women during pregnancy
  - Usually referenced as a tenfold increased risk from pregnancy
- Forty to sixty-five women out of 10,000 healthy women in the first three months **after** pregnancy
  - *Highest risk group is postpartum*, meaning after giving birth

Treatment:

The first step is diagnosis, but know that the answers are often more gray than black and white.

- Blood test: D-Dimer is a test that, if low or negative, can reassure us that there is no clot. An elevated D-Dimer does not confirm presence of a clot, but it does mean we need further investigation, including some type of imaging.
  - Many campus clinics can check D-Dimers but then must transfer the student to an emergency room for the next level of diagnostic tests.
- Duplex ultrasound: noninvasive test to look for clots in leg or arm veins.
- Additional imaging at hospitals may include chest scans or dyes injected into veins.

Once a blood clot is confirmed in your leg, arm, or lung, the treatment will be blood thinners (which may be given via IV, injection, or in pill form, with type, treatment length, and follow-up all dependent upon the size and location of your clot, as well as the rest of your medical history).

Head to your doctor if:

- You feel short of breath or are breathing too fast (more than twenty breaths per minute).
- Your heart is racing for no reason.

- You have unexplained chest pain.
- You have unexplained arm or leg pain, redness, or swelling.

Worst-case scenario:

Blood clots, especially those that travel to the lung, are potentially **lethal.**
Common? Thankfully not. ***But they are serious, so we don't want to miss a single one.***

Prevention:

- **Stop smoking** (or don't start!).
  - **What about vaping?** Right now, we have very few quality studies that purely address vaping, but obviously vaping has high concentrations of **nicotine**, which definitely **does** increase your risk of clots, heart attacks, and strokes. Don't vape.
  - **What about weed?** *Do we really need to go here?* Again, not legal long enough for excellent studies, but we know pot has negative cardiovascular effects. Lots of reasons to avoid cannabis products, so add this to the list.
- If you are in an all-day study session at a computer, set an alarm for short breaks every one to two hours and get up to walk for five minutes.
- Before a long flight, take an aspirin (its blood-thinning ability prevents clot formation) and consider compression travel socks. During the flight, make sure to get up and walk in the aisle (head to the bathroom) every couple of hours.

TIPS:

- ○ **Chest Pain or Shortness of Breath + Birth Control Pills = Potentially Serious Problem (Until Proven Otherwise!)** *We'd rather see a thousand students with symptoms who do NOT have a pulmonary embolism than miss one person who has this problem.*
- ○ *Pregnancy* increases your risk of developing a blood clot by a factor of ten (occurring in 1/1000 pregnancies, and more

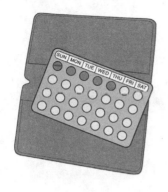

commonly than that in the first twelve weeks after giving birth), while *birth control pills* increase your risk by a factor of two to six. **Take-home message: For a nonsmoking, otherwise healthy, sexually active young woman, fear of clots should not cause you to avoid taking the pill.** Also, there are other nonhormonal choices of contraception if you have other risk factors.

○ The increased risk of clotting is also true for Nuvaring (the vaginal form of birth control) as well as Orthoevra (the birth control patch)—it's the estrogen, not the delivery method.

Chapter 37
Food Poisoning? Nausea, Vomiting, and Diarrhea

What If: I Get Food Poisoning?

Medical Name: Gastroenteritis

What most likely happened:

You felt fine all day, then a few hours after dinner, your stomach didn't feel quite right. Later while attempting to study, your uneasy gut erupted into full-blown nausea and vomiting that came in waves that kept you up for the rest of the night, worsened by progressively intense abdominal cramping and diarrhea. By morning, you are weak, lightheaded, seeing spots when you try to stand up, and every time you try to sip on water or Gatorade, it comes right back up.

What's going on?

Is this food poisoning or a stomach virus? *Does it matter?* Honestly, for your individual treatment, probably **not.** The cause is usually irrelevant, *because the primary treatment is rehydration, rest, and time.* Antibiotics are **rarely** required for nausea/vomiting/diarrhea illnesses, even when the cause is food poisoning.

For community health reasons, we try to identify clusters of outbreaks and their common source—so yes, we will ask where you've been eating the past day or two. If we see numerous students within a short time frame who all report eating the same type of food or at the same dining location, it's time to investigate. However, the onset of symptoms after eating contaminated food varies tremendously, making it challenging to figure out the cause for each individual.

- If you're vomiting **now**, the problem could be from a contaminated potato or egg salad a couple of hours ago (*Staph* poisoning—symptom onset at one to six hours), infected raw produce the day before yesterday (*norovirus*—symptoms starting in twelve to twenty-four hours), a burger last week (E.coli 0157:H7—symptoms begin after one to eight days), or long-forgotten oysters last month (*hepatitis A*—symptoms starting in fifteen to fifty days).
- **Viral infections** (like *norovirus,* a.k.a. cruise ship virus) remain the most common cause of food-borne illness in the United States, and this germ is crazily infectious, ripping through classrooms and dorms. If your roommate was sick yesterday and your suitemates were ill the day before, good chance it's a *norovirus* (which may be transmitted via food, person to person, or from touching your mouth after touching an infected surface). Remember COVID-19 can also show up as primarily gastrointestinal symptoms. A 2023 study showed patients started their illness with lack of appetite (21.2%), nausea (17.3%), vomiting (16.2%), and diarrhea (15.5%).
- **Bacterial food poisoning** in an otherwise healthy college student with mild to moderate symptoms *usually does not require antibiotics*, and in some cases, antibiotics can worsen the illness (such as with *hemorrhagic E. coli* or *non-typhoid salmonella*).
- **Giardia infection** deserves special mention because we do treat this diarrheal illness with antibiotics. The hallmark symptoms are prolonged (often more than a week) excessive gas (with

abdominal cramping and very smelly farting), nausea, and greasy, floating, or watery diarrhea. Giardia symptoms begin a week or two after exposure, and although this parasite can be transmitted through food (by infected food handlers with poor hand-washing hygiene), college students may be more likely infected via swimming (and accidentally ingesting contaminated water) in pools, streams, and lakes.

Ultimately, diagnosis for gastroenteritis is typically presumptive, based on your symptoms and potential exposure time line. Since most gastro-intestinal illnesses resolve on their own within a day or two, additional testing is rarely recommended, and even then, stool cultures identify the source less than half of the time. By the way, "stomach flu" does not mean influenza but is simply another way to say gastroenteritis/GI bug.

Treatment:
- Rehydration, time, and rest (and, very rarely, antibiotics)
- Antinausea medication
  - Ondansetron (Zofran) most commonly prescribed

How to REHYDRATE:
- Steadily sip on water, ice chips, frozen popsicles, or a sport beverage, **without** a straw (because straws introduce air into your stomach, potentially worsening nausea/vomiting).
- Avoid excess sugar (which can actually worsen diarrhea) by diluting full-calorie sport drinks with additional water.
- Rehydration solutions (like Pedialyte) include salt, sugar, and water in varying amounts; the "home brew" is mixing ½ teaspoon salt, 6 teaspoons sugar, and 5 cups of clean water.

Don't worry about eating food right away, but when you do eat, start with small amounts and avoid dairy and fatty foods. The traditional BRAT diet (bananas, rice, applesauce, toast) is fine to start reintroducing foods, but there's no need to stick exclusively to those foods.

Avoid caffeine, nicotine, alcohol, and antihistamines (allergy medications) because you are already dehydrated, and these substances will dehydrate you further, worsening your symptoms.

Antibiotics are considered when you have:
- High or persistent fever
- Severe symptoms
- Blood in the stool
- Symptoms that last beyond a week
- Traveler's diarrhea
- A job in health care, childcare, or food industry

Should you stop the diarrhea?
- Definitely **not** if you see blood in your stool
- *Though not generally encouraged,* if you have purely watery stools without blood (and no fever), symptoms *may* be helped with:
    - Antimotility medications like loperamide (Imodium)
    - Antisecretory medications like bismuth subsalicylate (Pepto-Bismol)
    - Antigas medications like simethicone (Gas-X)

What about Probiotics?
Probiotic supplements (yogurt, pills, powders) with lactobacilli or saccharomyces have been shown to help infectious diarrhea resolve faster in children, but the evidence is less definitive in adults. Bottom line? *They might help, but not a strong recommendation.*

Head to your doctor if you:
- Cannot keep down fluids.
- See blood in your stool.
- Have fever (temp greater than 100.5°F).
- Have diarrhea that persists more than a few days.
- Have recently taken an antibiotic.
- Have recently traveled to another country.
- Work in childcare, health care, or food service industry.

Worst-case scenario:

Usually the worst-case scenario is severe dehydration that requires IV fluids to rehydrate you (which can typically be done at your university clinic). Before starting IVs, though, we will try an antinausea medication that can be melted under your tongue (ondansetron, brand-name Zofran), and often even one dose will do the trick, allowing you to keep down oral fluids and avoid needing an IV.

Very rarely, food poisoning toxins or bacteria will persist, causing serious damage such as kidney failure (hemorrhagic *E. coli)* or miscarriage (*Listeria*) in a pregnant woman. Additionally, *Campylobacter* food poisoning has been identified as a trigger for Guillain-Barre syndrome, a rare neurological syndrome that induces a potentially life-threatening rapid paralysis.

Prevention:

Hand washing (*with soap for at least twenty seconds*) remains the best prevention for spread of these GI germs.

Dorm Food precautions:
- **Eat cooked leftovers (including pizza) within three days or throw away.**
- Always rinse fresh produce under running water (unless removing the skin before eating).
- Don't eat raw eggs (sorry, this means cookie dough and cake batter).
- Don't eat refrigerated foods that have sat out for longer than two hours (or longer than one hour if outside temp is hotter than 90°F).
- Opened deli meats are only good for three to five days.

TIPS:

- **Cleaning up vomit** (and poop) is critical to avoid spreading stomach illnesses! Often the symptoms come on with so little warning (or with such force) that you may end up with a mess.

- **Do NOT flush vomit down the sink** if you threw up there (that will clog the sink, too).
- Use disposable gloves or dog-poop bags to grab the big chunks (gross but accurate, sorry!) or just scoop out the vomit with generous amounts of paper towels into some other type of trash bag that you can immediately tie off and throw away in an outside dumpster. Then use a bleach-based cleaning spray on the sink, leave it on for a few minutes, then wipe off.
  - ➢ Note that bleach will actually **bleach**, leaving white spots if used on carpet or bedding.
- Finally, wash potentially contaminated clothes, towels, and bedding with detergent (in a washing machine).
- **Medications:**
  - Be aware that you may have thrown up any routine medications such as **birth control** and take appropriate precautions.
  - If you've thrown up multiple times, do not take any "as-needed" medications until you are keeping down plenty of fluids and at least some food; this includes ADHD medications and antihistamines (which will aggravate your symptoms and further dehydrate you).
- **Avoid consuming any dairy products for several days** after a diarrheal illness, because these infections frequently damage the superficial lining of your gut (where the lactase enzyme lives), thus making you *temporarily lactose intolerant* until the lining regenerates.
  - The most common cause of prolonged abdominal cramping and diarrhea after gastroenteritis is reintroduction of dairy too soon (aggravated by the myth that milk "soothes" your stomach).

Chapter 38
Public Restroom Panic—I Just Can't Go (Constipation)

What If: I Can't Poop?
Medical Name: Constipation

What most likely happened:
A couple weeks into your freshman year, you began noticing progressive abdominal bloating and discomfort, and frankly, it's gotten more and more difficult to have a bowel movement. You used to poop nearly every day, and now it's maybe twice per week. When you do poop, it looks like rabbit pellets with separate hard lumps. And how embarrassing is it to be in an elevator or small classroom or dorm room and be suffering from gas pains and smelly farts? Now you're stuck with frequent abdominal pain (or at least discomfort), and you don't know how to fix it.

What's going on?
Moving into a dorm where you share a bathroom with anywhere from four to forty others presents multiple challenges. Whether it's a large, multi-stall facility down the hallway in a dorm, or simply a suite-style bathroom

shared with a few others, the fear of others hearing your bodily noises or, heaven forbid, smelling the results can paralyze some people to the point that they . . . refuse to poop. Or uncomfortably hold it till they can find an empty bathroom in another building. Dehydration from poor water intake or excess caffeine only makes things worse, and weekend alcohol doesn't help at all. Additionally, the standard college diet is rich in pizza and burgers but notoriously lacking in fruits, veggies, and fiber, creating the perfect recipe for stopped-up bowels.

Dietary and situational constipation are very common, especially in the college setting. However, contributing factors may also include:

- **Metabolic problems:**
  - Hypothyroidism
  - Pregnancy
  - Diabetes
  - Hyperparathyroidism
- **Medications:**
  - Antihistamines
  - Antidepressants
  - Pain medications
  - Multivitamins (especially with iron)
  - Antiseizure medications
  - Calcium channel blockers (used to prevent migraines or high blood pressure)
  - Antacids (that contain aluminum)

Treatment:

If the primary issue is fear of public toileting, *this must be addressed first!* Know that this is a very common anxiety (an estimated 7 percent of the population), but if your level of public restroom avoidance is impacting your life to the point that you avoid social or academic gatherings, or causing abdominal discomfort because you consciously choose not to use certain bathrooms, then please, talk with your doctor or a counselor trained in CBT (Cognitive Behavioral Therapy) because we can help!

Toilet anxiety may also be purely a **fear of germs**, most commonly the specific fear of catching a sexually transmitted disease (STD). *Rest assured, the only way you will catch an STD in a public restroom is if you are having unprotected sex in that stall!* Seriously, there are **no** (**none, zilch, nada, zero**) STDs that are passed person to person from sitting down on a toilet seat. If the seat is wet with some unknown substance (more often water that splashes up, but certainly also urine), use toilet paper and wipe it dry because that's gross, but STDs are not going to enter your body through intact skin on the back of your legs as you sit on the seat.

Toilet anxiety can also be **a fear of bodily sounds and odors**. If this is your issue in a dorm suite situation, crank up your iTunes and keep a bottle of *Poo-Pourri* (or your favorite brand of bathroom odor stabilizer) on the back of the tank (plus a travel-sized bottle in your backpack for other bathrooms). If you are waiting in line in a public bathroom and people are "stuck" in the stalls, be that kind soul who decides to wash their hands and hope for a powerful hand blow dryer to create noise distraction.

Again, CBT can help you work through thought distortions you may have developed. Everyone poops, and everyone makes different noises as they defecate, causing varying degrees of transient embarrassment. Most people ignore it or laugh for a second but then immediately forget about other people's "noise." If you can't shake the unwanted, automatic thought "OMG, what will my friend/classmate/coworker/stranger think if they hear me?" then part of your treatment is learning to recognize and identify that **this is your thought**, *not a fact*. You cannot read minds, and you are likely catastrophizing.

Treatment

Treatment for constipation should begin with: **Water, Fiber, and Movement.**

- **Water:** Carry a large (25-ounce) water bottle in your backpack and drink at least two per day
  - Pro tip: if you don't need to pee every few hours, you are not drinking enough.

194

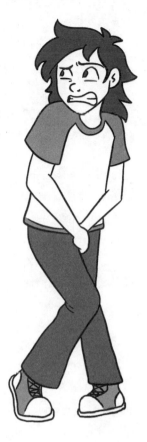

- **Fiber:** Goal is **20 to 25 grams of fiber** per day, and the best source is food (not powder supplements)
    - Consider high-fiber breakfast cereal (All-Bran Buds: 13 grams for ⅓ cup; Fiber One: 8 grams for 1 cup)
    - Snack on high-fiber granola bars (NuGo:12 grams per bar; KIND: 7grams perbar; Fiber One: 9 grams per bar)
    - **Add at least one fruit or vegetable to each meal:**
        - Banana: 3 to 4 grams
        - Pear (with skin): 6 grams
        - Apples (with skin): 4.4 grams
        - Raspberries (1 cup): 8 grams
        - Dried Plums (or prunes, 1 cup): 12 grams! (*Yes, that's why prunes "work"*)
        - Green peas (1 cup): 9 grams
        - Broccoli (1 cup): 5 grams
        - Carrots (1 cup): 4 grams
        - Sweet Potato (1 yam): 6 grams
- **Movement:** Get walking! The less mobile you are, the less your guts move food through. Exercise helps food pass through your large intestine more quickly, which means your stool holds on to more water and is therefore less hard and dry.

If you are doing all of the above and are still constipated, a laxative is the next step.

OTC products include:
- Osmotics like Milk of Magnesia or Miralax
- Stimulants like Dulcolax or Senekot

- Stool softeners like Colace or Surfak

Prescription Medications for your physician to consider:
- linaclotide (Linzess)
- lubiprostone (Amitiza)
- lactulose (Enulose)

Diagnostic testing such as blood work, abdominal imaging (ultrasound, X-ray, or CT scan), or even endoscopy may be ordered to rule out another medical disorder contributing to your constipation, but the majority of constipation treatment focuses on the behavioral changes above.

Head to your doctor if:
- You see blood in your stool.
- You develop severe pain, fever, or unintentional weight loss.
- Fear of public toileting is causing your constipation.
- OTC laxatives and dietary changes don't help after a week.

Worst-case scenario:
In otherwise healthy young people, the most common worst-case scenario of constipation is hemorrhoids, which show up as rectal discomfort, itching, a palpable bump, and/or bright red blood streaks in your stool. Prolonged sitting on the toilet with straining to poop causes rectal veins to dilate, which creates the hemorrhoid. Treatment includes topical steroid creams to help the rectal symptoms and, more important, treatment to improve the constipation that caused the hemorrhoids.

Prevention:
Water, fiber, and movement (see pages 194–195!)

TIPS:
- Antihistamines (Claritin, Allegra, Zyrtec, Benadryl) are very drying and a common contributor to constipation. If you need these meds for your allergies, double your water intake.

○ Normal frequency of bowel movements varies from twice a week to several times per day; constipation is therefore relative—what's important is a change from **your** normal pattern to far less frequent stools and/or hard/painful stools.

○ If you see bright-red blood in the toilet (or on the toilet paper) when you poop, don't freak out! Yes, you definitely should be examined by a doctor, but it's most likely an annoying hemorrhoid or small tear in your rectum, *not something scary like cancer.*

Chapter 39
Is My Stomach Pain Appendicitis?

What If: My Bad Stomachache Is My Appendix About to Rupture?

Medical Name: Appendicitis

What most likely happened:

Last night, your stomach felt "off," and all day today you have had no appetite at all . . . which basically never happens! After your last class, you trudged back across campus to your dorm room and crawled into bed. You feel mildly nauseated, no diarrhea or vomiting (yet), and your entire belly is bloated and aching, especially down low on the right side. Your premed roommate sees your flushed face and hands you a thermometer to check for a fever, and sure enough your temperature is 100.8°F. Your lab partner was diagnosed with influenza, and although you got your flu shot, you're wondering if you ended up with a mild case of the flu. Meanwhile, your boyfriend texted that his cousin had these exact symptoms before his appendix burst, so he wants to pick you up and take you to the doctor. What should you do?

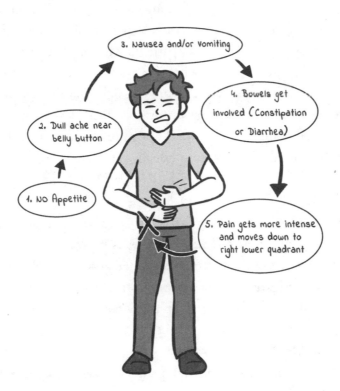

What's going on?

Appendicitis occurs in roughly 1 out of 1,000 Americans per year, but the majority of cases happen in ten-to-thirty-year-olds. As such, we see this with reasonable frequency in college students. The appendix lives in the lower right portion of your abdomen, a roughly 3½-inch skinny tube of tissue that extends out of your large intestine. When the opening to this tube is blocked by swelling, stool, or possibly seeds, the bacteria that always live in our gut rapidly multiply in a small space, creating local infection and inflammation. The danger is that if this rapidly swelling infection grows large enough to rupture the appendix, bacteria will spread throughout your entire abdomen, creating a potentially life-threatening infection.

Early on, it's tough to tell whether you've got a common stomach virus, food poisoning, or appendicitis. All may cause stomach pain, nausea, vomiting, bloating, diarrhea, or constipation. Certainly, if you have several other friends ill with the same symptoms, appendicitis is less likely.

Classic appendicitis pain starts off as a general ache in the center of your belly, then within four to twelve hours that pain sharpens and moves to your right lower belly. In practice, patients with appendicitis often think their whole stomach hurts, but when we examine them, it only hurts (or greatly intensifies the pain) when we are pressing over the appendix in that right lower area. This tenderness on exam, plus a fever and an elevated white blood cell count, point toward appendicitis, and typically the next step is an ultrasound or CT scan to visualize that area.

Treatment:

The primary treatment for appendicitis is surgical removal of the appendix, coupled with IV antibiotics. The good news is most appendicitis surgeries are done through a scope, so scars are minimal and recovery is quick. Trials continue to investigate whether antibiotics alone are a treatment option; downside is a high recurrence rate (up to 39 percent within five years).

Head to your doctor if you have:
- Fever and increasing stomach pain, *especially if pain moves to your right lower abdomen.*
- Abdominal pain and inability to pass gas or have a bowel movement.

Worst-case scenario:

As mentioned above, the worst case is a ruptured appendix that spreads infection throughout your abdomen; this requires prolonged IV antibiotics and most likely an open surgery not done through scopes, so larger incision and scar and longer recovery.

Prevention:

Although a high-fiber diet rich in fruits and vegetables may slightly lower your risk, the only way to prevent appendicitis is if your appendix has been surgically removed (because you had appendicitis previously, or it was removed during another abdominal surgery).

TIPS:

- There are no absolutes in medicine, but **if you are hungry** along with abdominal pain, bloating, and fever, *appendicitis is much less likely.*

- An uncomplicated laparoscopic appendectomy will leave you tired and sore for about a week, but the good news is that, if necessary, you can likely attend classes again within a day or two—although you will probably need to lighten up your backpack because you should not lift more than ten pounds this first week after your operation.

- **Sharp stomach pain is not limited to your appendix.** Other relatively common sources include gallstone pain (classically on the right upper part of your abdomen; pain comes in long, intense twenty-to-thirty-minute waves, runs in families), inflammation of the pancreas (from gallstones or heavy alcohol use), gastritis (from alcohol, nicotine, and anti-inflammatory medicine like ibuprofen), and pain referred upward (from ruptured ovarian cysts).

Chapter 40

College Is Giving Me Heartburn . . . or Maybe an Ulcer

What If: I'm Getting Heartburn . . . or Maybe an Ulcer?

Medical Name: Gastritis, Ulcers, and Gastroesophageal Reflux (GERD)

What most likely happened:

Your crazy stress over that calculus class has your stomach tied in knots, especially in the evenings. Meals leave you bloated, aching, and nause- ated, and sometimes your chest feels tight, too. Although you're pretty sure coffee won't help your stomach, your brain needs the caffeine to power through tonight's stack of practice tests . . . so you order a latte rather than your usual Starbucks. What else can you do?

What's going on?

Ulcers and heartburn have overlapping symptoms of upper abdominal pain, bloating, and worsening of symptoms after a meal. Ulcer symptoms typically stay focused south of your breastbone, and the pain is often more intense, possibly waking you up at night. With heartburn, however, you may also have burning pain in your chest, regular burping, "wet burps" where acid goes up to your mouth, sore throat, or trouble swallowing.

While stress doesn't directly cause ulcers or heartburn, many **coping habits** absolutely irritate the stomach lining, causing inflammation (gastritis) that promotes the development of ulcers along with acid reflux.

- **Alcohol**—especially with binge-drinking (quantity counts!)
- **Ibuprofen** (and other Anti-Inflammatory Drugs like aspirin, naproxen)
- **Nicotine** (traditional or e-cigs)
- **Caffeine**—though not clearly linked to gastritis, definitely causes heartburn. Acid is normally contained in the stomach by a muscular band of tissue (the lower esophageal sphincter) that closes after food and drink pass through. Caffeine, nicotine, and alcohol all relax this sphincter, which allows acid to then slosh back up into the esophagus. (This is why when people are uncomfortably full after eating a large meal, they may seek relief from a cocktail, coffee, or cigarette.)

Treatment:

For occasional heartburn, taking OTC antacids like TUMS, Rolaids, or Mylanta can immediately and directly neutralize your stomach acid.

For more frequent heartburn, consider a longer-acting OTC medicine that will decrease the production of stomach acid:

- **H2-Blockers**: cimetidine (Tagamet HB), famotidine (Pepcid AC), or nizatidine (Axid AR)
- **Proton Pump Inhibitors (PPIs)**: omeprazole (Prilosec) and lansoprazole (Prevacid)

If your gastritis progresses all the way to an ulcer, you'll need more than acid medications. Why? Because the vast majority of stomach ulcers are actually caused by *H. Pylori*, bacteria that live in the GI tracts of 30 percent of Americans. Treatment regimens vary but should include two antibiotics along with a long-acting acid-blocking medication for ten to fourteen days.

Head to your doctor if:
- You're taking antacids or acid-blocking pills multiple times per week.
- Your stomach pain is persisting or getting worse.
- You have trouble swallowing.
- You have nausea or vomiting.
- Your bowel movements become dark black (this may indicate blood in your stool).

Worst-case scenario:

The vast majority of reflux and gastritis symptoms can be diagnosed and managed by your primary care physician, but worst case is typically that you end up needing an endoscopy by a gastroenterologist to assess reflux or gastritis symptoms that do not improve with prescription medications.

Prevention:
- Drink alcohol (if you choose to do so) in moderation.
- Never smoke or vape.
- Avoid large meals, especially in the evening.

TIPS:
- Avoid clothing with tight waistbands.
- If your reflux mainly bothers you at night, try elevating the head of your bed by about six inches (consider a wedge pillow).
- Use acetaminophen (Tylenol) instead of ibuprofen (Advil/Motrin) or aspirin.
- If you live on breath mints, cut back or switch to gum; spearmint and peppermint candies or oils can worsen reflux.

Chapter 41

My Back (Pack) Is Killing Me

What If: My Back Is Killing Me?

Medical name: Low Back Pain/Strain

What most likely happened:

For several days or weeks, you've been noticing some discomfort and occasional spasm in your lower back on the right. This morning, you can barely get out of bed because the pain is so intense, and it's dramatically worse when you try to move in any direction. The pain is not extending down your legs or into your hips, but especially when you move, the pain shoots up the middle of your back toward one shoulder.

What's going on?

Low back pain in college students is often directly related to overly heavy backpacks that are carried incorrectly, creating strained muscle mechanics that trigger back muscle spasm.

Treatment:

- Basic initial treatment for muscular low back pain includes over the counter (OTC) medications such as NSAIDs (Nonsteroid

Anti-Inflammatory Drugs) like ibuprofen (brand names Advil, Motrin) plus the pain reliever acetaminophen (Tylenol). These two medications may be taken separately or together to relieve pain.

- **Moist heat**: a shower, a bath, or a moist-heat heating pad will help relieve spasm.
  - **Moist heat is better than ice therapy for the first five days.**
- For severe spasm, your doctor may prescribe muscle relaxant medications for short-term use, but since they are sedating, brain-fogging, and potentially addictive, we try to limit them to just a few days, taken only at bedtime.
- **Physical therapy**: including topical modalities like ultrasound and therapeutic massage, plus stretching and resistance exercises.
- Some people find relief from **OTC topical creams or pads** that contain counterirritants like menthol or oil of evergreen; these products create a cooling or burning sensation that distracts from pain (e.g., Icy Hot, Salonpas pads).

Head to your doctor if:
- You have **severe pain or intense spasm** that limits your movement.
- You have **back pain with fever** or any **urinary symptoms** (likely not muscular back pain).
- You have **back pain that radiates** down through your buttocks or into your legs.

Worst-case scenario:
Though significantly less common in college-aged young adults, occasionally people rupture or herniate a disc in their back, causing sciatica (nerve pain that shoots down into the leg) and other complications.

Prevention:
- The **maximum weight** you should routinely carry is **20 percent of your body weight**, and *ideally, you should limit it to 10 percent of your body weight.*

- **Invest in a lightweight backpack** with cushioned shoulder straps and back padding and try to consistently use **both** straps—do **not** sling over one shoulder.
- **Lighten up** your backpack:
  - Opt for e-books whenever possible.
  - Use a tablet (such as an iPad) with a keyboard case instead of a laptop.
- If you must use one shoulder, at least **alternate shoulders** every five to ten minutes and/or intermittently carry the pack with both arms in front of your body.
- If your backpack is heavier than usual, **use the chest and hip straps** as well, *at least while you are riding your bike to class.*
- **Avoid bending over** when you are wearing a backpack—bend your knees and squat if you have to pick something up (or take off the backpack first).
- **Core strengthening and stretching** through basic exercises or yoga can improve posture and muscle mechanics to help prevent low back pain.

TIPS:

- o **Weigh your loaded backpack!** (Max weight should be 10 to 20 percent of your weight.)
- o **If you live off campus** and need to carry "everything" with you each day, **lighten up when you arrive:** unload what heavy items you don't need for the first half of the day into a secure cubby, study room, locker, or friend's dorm room, then swap out midday.

○ **When your back HURTS:**

  ○ **Keep moving**—bed rest is **not** the answer! Staying active promotes faster healing, so get out and walk rather than hibernating in bed.

  ○ When you do sleep, position yourself on your side with a pillow placed between your bent knees. If you also have a "body pillow," prop that behind your body to keep you from rolling over to your back.

○ **If you have back pain without any specific injury** (such as a bad fall or a car, bike, or scooter accident), ***do not expect an X-ray***: imaging is *rarely* indicated for acute low back pain, and the radiation does you no favors.

Chapter 42

My Double-Over Back (or Side) Pain Is a Kidney Stone

What If: My Double-Over Back or Side Pain Is a Kidney Stone?

Medical Name: Nephrolithiasis

What most likely happened:

Yesterday (or all weekend), you were studying all day in the library, drinking only coffee to stay awake. *(Feel free to insert any way to get dehydrated, such as "Yesterday I drank too much beer while sweating all day at a scorching-hot SEC football game.")* After going to bed, you woke up feeling a vague back, side, or abdominal discomfort, and then suddenly you had double-over stabbing pain in one spot that vice-gripped you for twenty minutes to an hour. As the pain finally eased, mild nausea and chills set in, and you wondered if you were getting the flu. Heading to the bathroom, you might have some trouble or discomfort urinating, see blood in your urine, or notice your urine is cloudy or smells bad. *Or you might not notice anything unusual at all about your urine.*

209

Then . . . the pain returns, and the cycle repeats: intense pain often paired with bad nausea and/or vomiting, lasting for twenty or more minutes that seem like a lifetime, and then slowly easing. Kidney stone pain comes in intermittent tidal waves, as the stone is slowly pushed down the tube (ureter) running from your kidney to your bladder.

However, the waves are so long that often people try medicine like TUMS or ibuprofen during the pain, and then the pain seems to improve, making it appear that the medicine is helping. When the pain returns, people repeat what "helped" before, and so on. In retrospect, it seems obvious that you had waves or cycles of pain, but when you are experiencing it, the big picture is much less clear. Also, while classically the painful spot slowly moves down your body, correlating with the stone's downward progression, not all stones **can** move, so some kidney stone pain sticks in one spot.

What's going on?

Kidney stones occur in one in eleven adults in the United States, with white males having the highest incidence. Since these stones are uncommon before age twenty, *college students with kidney stones are often experiencing their first stone* and therefore often have no idea what is going on, unless they've seen a family member or friend suffer through one.

Urine is filled with chemicals that can potentially crystallize, like calcium, urate, oxalate, phosphate, and xanthine. In a well-hydrated, healthy kidney, these substances are flushed out and don't have time to bind together to form crystals. However, in certain situations when risk factors combine, a stone is formed that may enlarge to the point of getting stuck as it passes downstream. Fortunately, despite the often-excruciating pain of passing a kidney stone, little or no actual damage is done to your urinary tract, and about 85 percent of stones will pass spontaneously (90 percent of stones are less than 6mm, whereas 59 percent of stones are greater than 6mm).

Do I need an X-ray?

Especially if this is your first kidney stone, your clinician will likely order some type of imaging, but probably not a regular X-ray. Ultrasound offers the advantages of lower cost and no radiation but is less accurate than a CT scan.

Why scan? To see the number, size, and location of your stone(s), as well as to assess the size of the kidney and whether the stone is fully obstructing the flow of urine.

You have a higher risk of getting kidney stones if you are (or have):

- Male
- White
- Obese
- Diabetic
- Heavy consumption of tea and sodas
- Gout
- Work/Live in a hot environment (so you are often dehydrated)
- Family members who have had kidney stones

HOWEVER: you may have NONE of these risk factors and still get kidney stones!

Treatment:

- Initial treatment is hydration and pain management. If you are not too nauseated to drink, then steadily sip on water or any noncaffeinated, nonalcoholic beverage, which will ultimately create more urine and help flush the stone downstream.
- If you are unable to drink enough fluids, IV fluids are the best way to speed fluid into your system.
- Antinausea medications like ondansetron (Zofran) can help decrease your nausea to allow you to drink more fluids.
- Nonsteroid Anti-Inflammatory Drugs (NSAIDs) like oral ibuprofen and injectable prescription ketorolac (Toradol) are the preferred medications to manage kidney stone pain.
- For larger stones (greater than 5mm), clinicians may add on another medication (an alpha-blocker) to help relax and dilate the ureters, thus making a larger, easier passageway for your stone.

- Treatment is not complete without giving you a urine strainer to hopefully capture your stone, in order to determine what specific type of stone your body produced:
    - Calcium oxalate (most common)
    - Uric acid (second place)
    - Struvite (caused by certain infections)
    - Cystine (uncommon, with a genetic predisposition)

Note that you are not looking for a grape- or even a pea-sized stone! Stones are much smaller than you think (and feel), with most appearing like a tiny fragment of gravel, around 1 to 3mm.

Head directly to your doctor if:
- Your pain is severe.
- Nausea or pain prevents you from drinking fluids.
- You cannot urinate.
- You see blood in your urine.
- You pass a kidney stone, then have new or worsening urinary symptoms.
    - Stones increase your risk of urinary tract infection.

Worst-case scenario:

Some stones are too large to pass on their own, and some create an obstruction that can damage the kidney and completely block the flow of urine on that side. Treatment options include shock-wave lithotripsy (using sound waves to break up larger stones) and surgical intervention (sliding a scope up through the urethra and bladder or directly inserting instruments through the skin to break up or remove a stone).

Prevention:
- **Hydration, hydration, hydration!** The more you can drink noncaffeinated, noncarbonated beverages, the better, with a goal of two to three liters per day. Remember that caffeine and alcohol

are diuretics, meaning they make you urinate **more**, so they are **dehydrating** agents, not a source of hydration.

- The type of stone you had, along with a twenty-four-hour urine collection analysis, will further direct dietary recommendations and supplemental medications that may help you prevent recurrent stones.

TIPS:

○ Though kidney stone pain is often severe, some people experience only mild discomfort, and pain is not directly proportionate to the size of the stone.

○ If you have **no symptoms**, and kidney stones are discovered incidentally when you have an X-ray or CT scan for another issue, only 10 to 25 percent of those stones will end up causing a problem, so simply staying well hydrated may be the only treatment that you need.

○ If you have the most common type of stone—calcium oxalate— this does **not** mean that you need to cut calcium out of your diet. In fact, low calcium diets actually **increase** your risk of developing calcium oxalate stones!

    ○ Try to pair up high-calcium food or drinks (dairy or fortified juices) with high-oxalate foods (nuts, spinach, chocolate, and yams) so these substances bind together in your gut before they are absorbed and sent to the kidneys.

Chapter 43
UTIs: Kidney and Bladder Infections

What If: I Get a Bladder/Kidney Infection?

Medical Name: Urinary Tract Infection (UTI)

What most likely happened:

Scenario A: Midterms are approaching, which means marathon study sessions with too much caffeine. Two nights ago, it burned a bit when you had to pee before you left the library. Yesterday morning, it burned more, and you spent all day running back and forth to the bathroom, meanwhile trying to ignore your body because you don't have time to go to the clinic. Today it's worse—the burning, the urgent dash to the bathroom, and before you even wash your hands, it feels like you need to go again. On top of that, your stomach is getting queasy, your back is aching, and you're starting to feel feverish.

Scenario B: You're newly sexually active this year, and although you never had a single bladder infection before college, this is the third time in two months that you are dealing with UTI symptoms. What's up?

What's going on?

Simple geography explains why women get UTIs far more often than men: the female's pooping area (anus) is closer to her peeing place (urethra).

Bacteria from our intestines/feces (most commonly *E. coli*) migrate forward in a damp environment and enter the urethra, moving upstream to the bladder and possibly all the way up to the kidneys. Sex, especially without condoms, produces extra fluids that become a bacterial express lane to infection. Similarly, after using the restroom, "reverse" toilet paper wiping from back to front efficiently transports the bacteria straight to your urinary tract.

One way the urinary tract fights infection is by constantly flushing the system, literally washing the bacteria downstream and out of the body. Therefore, if you ignore your urge to empty your bladder and spend too many hours without a bathroom break, this allows your urine to stagnate and bacteria to multiply, setting the stage for a UTI. Or if you don't drink enough water, you can't make enough urine to do that necessary flushing. On the opposite end, drinking excessive amounts of caffeine directly irritates the bladder, which also makes you more likely to get a UTI.

Finally, cosmetic products such as douches or sprays advertised to cleanse your lady parts end up merely irritating your skin, vaginal tissue, and urethra, causing painful urination and possibly setting up a UTI. ***Our bodies are designed to cleanse themselves . . . just add water!***

Treatment:

- Simple bladder infections are easily treated with a short course of antibiotics.
- Kidney infections require stronger antibiotics and usually longer courses.
- For women who seem to develop UTIs virtually every time they have sex, physicians may offer "postcoital antibiotic prophylaxis," which is a prescription for a single dose of antibiotic to be taken each time after intercourse.
- Antibiotics can't work if you're not well hydrated, so drink plenty of water or **any** noncaffeinated, nonalcoholic liquid. (Caffeine and alcohol are diuretics that irritate the bladder.)

Head to your doctor if:
- You have urinary burning, frequency, or urgency.
- You have fever, chills, nausea, or vomiting along with any urinary discomfort.
- You develop back pain along with urinary discomfort.

Worst-case scenario:

A simple bladder infection can progress to a more serious kidney infection (pyelonephritis), which may require IV antibiotics, IV hydration, and hospitalization.

Prevention:

- **Drink. More. Water!**
- Women: pee after sex. You don't have to leap out of bed the second you finish, but don't fall asleep before you head to the restroom.
- If you are sexually active, use condoms, preferably with lubricant (less irritating to your skin/vagina/urethra).
- If you develop intercourse-related UTIs and are using a diaphragm and/or spermicide, talk to your doctor about different options for birth control (because diaphragms and spermicide increase your risk of UTIs).
- Women: after using the restroom, always wipe front to back one time, then drop the toilet paper in the toilet. If you need to wipe more, grab a few more sheets and repeat.
- Avoid bubble baths, bath oils, douching, and anything other than a mild soap and water to cleanse your pelvic area.

TIPS:

- **Azo Standard and Pyridium:**
  - **Warning**: Your urine will turn **bright red or orange**, terrifying unsuspecting users because it looks like **blood**.

- o Orange-stained urine messes up our quick, color-coded "dip stick" urine test, so unless you're miserable, wait until after your doctor's visit to start this type of pain reliever.

- o These OTC medications stop the burning pain of urination by numbing the urinary tract, but *you still need antibiotics to treat your infection.*

- o **Cranberry Juice?** Sure, drink it if you like it, but studies show that to make it more effective than water, you have to drink large amounts of 100 percent juice (not the cocktail versions), which is probably not worth the financial or caloric cost.

- o **If you are sexually active, burning with urination** may result from a sexually transmittable infection like chlamydia or gonorrhea, rather than from a basic bladder infection. **Get tested,** even if the symptoms go away after a day or two. This is especially true with guys, because healthy young males rarely get UTIs. But absolutely true for women, too! Why? *Because most STIs are silent or only cause transient symptoms.* Disappearing symptoms do not equal disappearing infection.

Chapter 44
The "Missing" Tampon

What If: My Tampon Disappeared?
Medical Name: Retained Tampon ("Foreign Body")

What most likely happened:
You head to the bathroom to change out your tampon, and . . . wait, what? Panic sets in as you search for the string without success. How can your tampon be missing? *(You would be surprised how often this happens.)* Most often, you simply don't remember removing your tampon because you were exhausted, totally preoccupied, or intoxicated. No big deal. However, at least a couple times per month, we find the missing tampon scrunched sideways, pushed up underneath the cervix, string and all, which is also usually not a big deal . . . *except the odor.*

What's going on?
Tampons that are "lost" and stuck for days create the perfect culture plate for local bacteria, which multiply like crazy, producing an offensive odor. Some women may not even realize they "lost" a tampon, only becoming concerned when they notice a vaginal discharge with a powerful smell. One of my favorite gynecologists, Lauren Streicher, MD, tells her triage nurse to ask, "Does it smell a bit fishy, or like the whole zoo?" If the answer is "the whole zoo," bet on a "lost tampon"!

Treatment:

Removal of the rogue tampon solves the problem, which is typically a simple, very quick procedure for your clinician because she has the benefit of using a speculum, which allows her to see where you cannot. If you are going to try removal yourself (which is often effective), be sure to wash your hands first (of course) or use a glove, and use your index and third fingers together to "grab" the edge and pull. Using one finger typically ends up merely pushing around the offending object, possibly shoving it farther out of your reach. (Rest assured, this is a limited space, so your clinician should definitely be able to find and retrieve anything left behind.) Depending on how long the tampon has been stuck and the degree of infection, your doctor may or may not also prescribe a topical or oral antibiotic (but most of the time, that is not necessary).

Head to your doctor:

Please do not wait! *If you are unsure of whether you accidentally left in a tampon or any other object you cannot find, schedule an appointment and let us look.* The longer you wait, the more you will suffer as you start having discharge, discomfort, and odor, and the greater risk you have of developing a more serious infection.

Worst-case scenario:

Tampons left in and ignored will cause a vaginal infection that can escalate, with the absolute very worst case being toxic shock syndrome (TSS). Toxic shock is caused by actual toxins from either staph or Strep bacteria, causing a rapid progression of high fever, headache, seizures, confusion, vomiting or diarrhea, sepsis, and potentially death.

Prevention:

- Proper, attentive use of tampons, changing them every four to six hours and never leaving one in for more than eight hours
- No matter how heavy your flow, use only one tampon at a time, with the lightest absorbency that works for your flow.

TIPS:

○ The exact same thing can happen with a condom (or a piece of a broken condom) that works its way off during sex.

○ Ditto for any other object placed in a vagina or anus.

○ If you think something **might** be stuck inside you, do NOT wait—go in and be seen as soon as possible! We've seen it before, and you won't be the last—don't let embarrassment keep you away.

○ Thinking of douching to flush it out or "cleanse" the area? Absolutely do NOT. That stuck tampon is now teeming with bacteria, and you certainly don't want to flush those infectious agents higher up into your genital tract!

    ○ Side note: The American Academy of Obstetricians and Gynecologists consistently reminds women that douching should not be a routine part of female hygiene, and in fact, douching is NEVER recommended. Vaginas are self-cleaning, with their own natural secretions and pH balance. Douching messes this up by changing the acidity and shifting the balance of the normal flora (bacteria), making you much more likely to develop vaginal dryness, irritation, and infections. Ditto for scented vaginal products, pads, and sprays. Just say no.

    ○ PS: Douching after sex is most assuredly NOT an effective means of birth control. In fact, douching potentially facilitates upstream access for the sperm, which is the opposite. Condoms, birth control pills, IUDs (and of course abstinence) prevent pregnancy; douching does NOT.

Chapter 45

Sexually Transmitted Infections (Yes, It Happens to People like You)

What If: I've Got a Bump/Blister/Discharge/ Itch "Down There"?

Medical Name: Sexually Transmitted Infection (STI)

What most likely happened:

Scenario A: You are newly sexually intimate with your first college boy-friend or girlfriend—in fact, only having oral sex, but now you've got a couple small patches of painful red blisters down there . . .

    Scenario B: College rocks! Your weekends have been so blissfully filled with parties and hookups—no strings attached—that last weekend you actually ran out of condoms. Best you can remember, you broke your self-imposed, previously ironclad rule and had sex at least once without protec-tion. Although it's hard to believe anyone in your friend group would have "that" kind of disease, given the worsening burning when you pee, plus seeing a small amount of discharge on your underwear, you're pretty sure you caught something.

Scenario C: You broke up with your long-term high school sweetheart last semester, and since then, you haven't been with anyone else, even though your friends bitterly report your "ex" has moved on to multiple new partners. Your birthday celebration last weekend was supposed to help you move on, but when your ex showed up, the combo platter of alcohol and overpowering old chemistry tossed you back in bed together. A week or two later (heart and pride still stinging from the insulting "morning-after" brush-off), you had a couple days of burning or irritation when you went to the restroom, but thankfully those symptoms disappeared, so you must be okay, right? Maybe you'll go get tested to be sure.

What's going on?

Sexually Transmitted Infections (STIs, also called STDs or Sexually Transmitted Diseases) are incredibly common, especially in young adults. Don't kid yourself that your college friends are too smart, rich, educated, religious, beautiful, or "whatever" to have herpes, chlamydia, genital warts, gonorrhea, HIV, or any other STI. Variations of the scenarios above are stories we hear every day in college health—*and I'm in urgent care, neither our women's health department nor the STD clinic.*

Scenario A: Herpes Simplex Virus (HSV). Understand herpes is **very common**! Roughly half of American adults ages fourteen to forty-nine are infected with HSV type 1 ("cold sore" herpes) whether or not they get cold sores, and one in five teens/young adults have genital herpes, which is caused by either HSV type 1 or HSV type 2. Think about this—if you have ten friends, on average, two are affected (but it could also be half or more of your friends, because obviously this virus does not line up and then uniformly distribute herpes to every fifth person across the planet). Note that the 27 percent of fourteen-to-nineteen-year-olds that already have "cold sore" oral HSV type 1 most likely got it from their families, from sharing drinks or nonsexual kissing. However, a large percentage of the new genital herpes cases that we see come from transmission of this "cold sore" herpes virus during oral sex, *regardless of whether the person performing oral sex currently has a visible cold sore.*

Scenario B: Bottom line . . . it only takes one time, *especially without a condom*, to contract an STI. Which one? In this setting of dysuria (painful urination) and discharge (whether you own a penis or a vagina), we anticipate that the most likely offenders are chlamydia and/or gonorrhea, both bacterial STIs that are happily curable with appropriate antibiotics. *Note that other STIs like trichomonas or even viral STIs including herpes, HPV, and HIV can also show up this way.*

What should you know about chlamydia and gonorrhea?

- Bacterial STIs that love to travel in packs; so commonly diagnosed together that if you test positive for gonorrhea, we automatically treat you for both gonorrhea and chlamydia.
- **Untreated**, both can lead to scarring in your reproductive tract, which can cause advanced infections (Pelvic Inflammatory Disease/ PID), chronic pain, and/or infertility.
- Gonorrhea has become a "superbug" that is resistant to the vast majority of antibiotics that used to easily eliminate it. *We do not mess around with this infection*—you will need both an antibiotic injection and oral antibiotics, plus a follow-up test to be **sure** we have cured you. Do **not** skip a single pill or the follow-up test, or you risk dealing with a super-SUPER bug that we might not be able to kill.
- Most of these infections are **silent**—no symptoms at all, till they've been marinating in your reproductive system long enough to scar and permanently damage your fertility.

Scenario C: Typically, nothing good comes from hooking up with an ex, particularly a long-term ex; remember the reason (or hundred reasons) why you broke up! Rebroken hearts and deflated self-images are often more difficult to fix than any STIs, but believe me, these are all very common outcomes. People in monogamous relationships rarely continue to use condoms, so when you reconnect with an old flame, hormones and emotions thrust you right back to your previous sexual relationship . . . without STI protection.

Lesson 1: If you are sexually intimate with *anyone (including your ex)*, use a barrier!

Lesson 2: STI symptoms are often fleeting and/or minimal; the only way to know if you are newly infected after an intimate encounter is to **get tested**.

Let's talk about SILENT STIs:
- 75 percent of females and 50 percent of males with chlamydia
- 30 percent of females and 10 percent of males with gonorrhea
- Majority of all people with HPV (Human Papilloma Virus)
- 20 percent of HIV infections
- Up to 90 percent of herpes simplex infections
- 90 percent of males with trichomonas infections

But if you have no symptoms, why does it matter? Because:

1. **Silent, untreated infections can progress in YOUR body**:
   a. Bacterial infections like gonorrhea and chlamydia can extend up your genital tract and cause damage and scarring that lead to chronic pelvic pain or infertility.
   b. HIV infection obviously affects the entire body and can progress to AIDS.
   c. Human Papilloma Virus (HPV) high-risk strains can cause cancer.
2. **Silent, untreated infections can be spread to your partners:**
   Minimal or no symptoms in you does not mean that same infection will be just as "weak" in your partner. Classic example is a mildly annoying genital herpes infection in one partner that becomes a frequently recurring, hugely painful, or frustrating infection in a partner.

Treatment:
- **Herpes:** An antiviral prescription medication (such as name-brands Acyclovir, Famvir, or Valtrex) may be prescribed for

each outbreak or taken daily as suppressive therapy to prevent outbreaks.

- **Chlamydia and Gonorrhea:** Combination treatment includes an injection of one antibiotic (ceftriaxone) in your hip plus one oral dose of azithromycin (antibiotic). Follow-up testing critical to ensure that your infection has cleared after treatment is key, as is avoiding reinfection from any untreated partners.
- **Human Papilloma Virus (HPV)—warts or cancer:** Prevention is easy with the HPV vaccine; but treatment is challenging.
  - Genital warts may be treated with a variety of creams, ointments, gels, acids, liquid nitrogen, or surgery; recurrence is very common.
  - HPV-related cervical, vulvar, anal, and throat cancer treatments include chemotherapy, surgery, and radiation.
- **Trichomonas:** Treatment includes a week-long course of an antibiotic, most commonly metronidazole (an antibiotic that can cause severe nausea and vomiting if you drink alcohol during the course of this prescription).
- **HIV:** Treatment involves multiple prescription medications to slow down this ever-evolving virus; but the good news is people are living full lives.

Head to your doctor:
- If your partner lets you know they've been diagnosed with an STI.
- If you have genital itching, burning, discharge, blisters, or bumps.
- If you've had a new partner, it's time to get tested. Period.

Worst-case scenario:

While we have over a million people living with HIV disease with all the medical and social challenges that this diagnosis includes, to me, the worst-case scenario is this: *preventable* future infertility. If you get a simple case of bacterial gonorrhea or chlamydia, we can **cure** this with a short course of antibiotics **IF** you get promptly diagnosed and treated. If you ignore the possibility that you could have one of these diseases, refusing testing for years and downplaying occasional symptoms, you may end up with scarring that leads to unwanted infertility.

Each year in the United States, we have close to 2 million reported confirmed cases of chlamydia and half a million cases of gonorrhea. Since most infections have no symptoms (and therefore people don't get tested), we know the real numbers are much higher, with an estimated 3.5 million total cases. Untreated, about 10 to 15 percent of these infections will progress to pelvic inflammatory disease (PID), and up to 20 percent of these women will develop tubal pregnancies, chronic pelvic pain, or infertility.

Prevention:

Obviously, if you **choose** not to be sexually active, your risk is zero (unless you were sexually assaulted). If you never drive or ride in a car, you don't have to worry about seat belts or car wrecks, because your risk is also zero. Enough said. However, if you do choose to be sexually active, using barriers (condoms/dental dams) 100 percent of the time will **dramatically** reduce your risk of contracting an STI and/or subsequent medical complications including chronic pelvic pain and/or infertility. Additionally, Frank Domino, MD, reminds us that *"hooking up is not just risky for STIs. Remember that assault can be one person's word against another, and you both need enthusiastic, nonintoxicated verbal consent. If you or your partner are drunk, stop. Don't do it."* (See Chapter 46: Date Rape and Sexual Assault, page 228.)

HPV VACCINE: Gardasil is extremely effective for both males and females. If you don't want cervical, penile, anal, or throat cancer, or genital warts—then get this vaccine before you are sexually intimate with another person.

Medications: Prescription antiviral medications can reduce your risk of contracting Herpes or HIV from an infected partner; talk to your doctor about options.

TIPS:
o Repeating louder for the people in the back row: **If you choose to be sexually intimate with oral, anal, or vaginal sex, Use. A.**

Condom. Every. Time. Yes, even with oral sex—get flavored condoms. No exceptions!!

○ One of the biggest mistakes is people assuming *if their symptoms go away, they are not infected* . . . but they are indeed infected. **Get Tested.**

○ Receptive anal intercourse (without a condom) is the highest risk/easiest way to catch an STI, because the anus lacks natural lubricant and the lining is more fragile (versus a vagina or mouth); friction easily creates tiny tears in the lining, allowing STIs easier access.

○ Women: unless you are taking an antibiotic **and** are not sexually active, *please do not assume vaginal irritation is a yeast infection*. If you have symptoms, get checked out.

○ **Young women are very fertile**! As a group, you do not have to work hard to conceive. In addition to using condoms to prevent STIs, heterosexual couples should be sure they have a second form of contraception (birth control pill, IUD, diaphragm, or another long-acting form of contraception).

○ **Basic STI testing is no big deal**—a urine test for chlamydia and gonorrhea, plus a blood test for HIV and syphilis. If you're mature enough to have sex, please do it responsibly by getting tested and knowing your (and your partner's) STI status.

○ Pubic lice ("crabs") are the single most contagious STI (nearly 100 percent transmission rate during sex), and, though far less often, these parasites can also be spread by infested clothing, bedding, or linens; avoid shared bedding and keep underwear on while trying on swimsuits.

○ *Can you catch an STI from a "virgin"?* Yes, because oral and anal sex can easily spread STIs, and opinions vary as to how these intimacies affect "virginity" status.

○ Public toilets do **not** spread STIs unless you are having sex in the stalls; stop worrying!

Chapter 46
Date Rape and Sexual Assault

What If: Date Rape?
Medical Name: Sexual Assault

What most likely happened:
Scenario A: Everything was going great with your date; in fact, better than you had hoped. The chemistry between you was amazing, and you were full-on *yes* . . . until things started to go too far, and you said *no*. But they didn't stop.

Scenario B: The last thing you remember was suddenly feeling super drunk and dizzy at the party. Now your head is throbbing, your stomach is churning, and half your clothes are on the floor of an unfamiliar room. Then aching down low tells you all you need to know—it happened to you.

What's going on?
Nearly a quarter (23 percent) of female and 5.4 percent of male undergraduates experience sexual assault through physical force or incapacitation, with the highest risk during the first year of college.

Any unwanted sexual contact (touching, oral sex, anal sex, or intercourse) without consent is sexual assault; rape refers specifically to penetration (oral, anal, or vaginal). Most sexual assaults are not between strangers; up to 90 percent of college students who have been assaulted know their attacker.

Treatment:

Most university health centers and virtually all hospitals offer a Sexual Assault Forensic Exam (SAFE, formerly known as a "rape kit" exam) that must be performed within four days of the assault, collecting evidence that will be preserved for two years while you decide whether to pursue criminal charges. *Having this exam does not require you to file charges, however.* Ideally, this exam should be done as soon as possible after the assault, and you should **not** clean up beforehand—don't change clothes, shower, brush your teeth, or wash or comb your hair (although if you've already done so, you can still have this exam).

Regardless of whether you choose a SAFE exam, you should be tested for sexually transmitted infections and, if appropriate, offered emergency contraception.

Counseling is critical—this was NOT YOUR FAULT, yet most victims blame themselves to some degree, especially if they were drunk, high, or perhaps even initiated the interaction. None of this matters; if you did not give consent, you were assaulted. And to be clear, assault is assault, regardless of gender or sexual preference. One more time because this is so important—***this is not your fault!***

Head to your doctor if:

You may have been or were sexually assaulted (*mind-altering substances often blur or erase details; do not hesitate to go in if you are concerned but unsure*).

Worst-case scenario:

The worst case here is that you tell no one and do not seek help. Sexually Transmitted Infections (STIs/STDs) and pregnancy can be prevented, diagnosed, and treated if you are seen as soon as possible. The biggest problem with STIs is that many are silent yet can still be passed on to others or do damage to your reproductive tract. Getting tested is the only way you will know for sure.

- See Chapter 45: Sexually Transmitted Infections (Yes, It Happens to People like You), starting on page 221.

Prevention:
- Choose a canned or bottled individual serving of alcohol that you open yourself (bottle of beer, individual serving wine bottle, or canned spritzer like White Claw) and never set down your drink.
- Frank Domino, MD, suggests if you don't want people to keep offering you drinks all night, ***"Start with a bottle of beer that is brown or green, then simply refill it with water. Only you will know what you are drinking."***
- Choose at least one designated nondrinking friend each night, *even if you are going to UBER,* so someone sober is making sure no one in your group leaves alone or gets too intoxicated.
- Make "escape" plans ahead of time with your friends, so if one of you feels uncomfortable, you all have a code word or phrase that lets the others know you want to leave, no questions asked. And if all else fails, "accidentally" spill your drink on yourself so you have to leave.

TIPS:
- Clear-headed (nonintoxicated), enthusiastic mutual *yes* means *yes* only when it is truly okay to say *NO*; nothing else is consent. Even then, remember that *yes* can change to *no* at any time for any reason.
- Even a slightly buzzed *yes* tonight may be a regret tomorrow, because intoxication at any level impairs judgment. Don't go there. **Intoxicated consent is not consent.**
- "Date rape" is a felony offense, no different from rape by a stranger.
- Alcohol remains the most common "date rape" drug, far more common than GHB, Rohypnol, or Ketamine.
- STI testing after sexual assault does not have to include a pelvic exam. Don't let that fear keep you from seeking care.

○ Gonorrhea, chlamydia, and trichomonas can be tested with urine samples, while HIV and syphilis require a blood sample.

○ Since some STIs will not show up immediately, testing should be repeated two weeks after the assault.

Chapter 47

Is It Broken? Toe, Wrist, and Stress Fractures

What If: It Might Be Broken?

Medical Name: Fracture

What most likely happened:

Scenario A: Ouch! Walking barefoot through your darkened dorm room, you jammed your toe against the metal bed frame so hard you saw stars. Next morning, you woke up to a painful, black-and-blue, swollen pinky toe, and you can barely walk on it.

  Scenario B: Racing late to class, you trip and fall forward on an outstretched hand. In addition to the embarrassment and road-rash on the heel of your hand, your wrist is aching . . . but you can wiggle all your fingers, so you assume you're fine. A few days pass, and your wrist is still swollen and sore, but there's not much bruising and you can still move your fingers. Should you go get examined?

  Scenario C: A service fraternity is sponsoring a half marathon, and your friends convince you to sign up a few weeks before the race. Though you've been less active in college, you played soccer (or danced, played volleyball/basketball, etc.) through high school; one thirteen-mile race seems doable. Dr. Google suggests a slower ramp-up on your training runs than you have time for, so you speed things up by doubling the recommended distance. By the third week, the front of your legs, especially your right leg, hurts with every run. The pain is better each morning, but even walking to class aches. When you press on it, there is one really tender spot along the inside front of your tibia, although you don't see any bruising or obvious swelling. Is this "just" shin splints or something more serious?

What's going on?

A. Toe and finger fractures are extremely common, especially in the college setting of intramural sports (jamming fingers catching balls) and darkened, unfamiliar, or overcrowded dorm rooms (especially with forced triples) with toe-stubbing hazards like bed risers and heavy desk edges. With a forced "jam" of a toe or finger, the flexor or extensor tendons can pull off small fragments of the middle or end bone, so the fracture in this case is often not a break through the whole bone, but a chip pulled off. Multiple fractures are common from one injury, especially with the "lesser" toes (not including the big toe). Particularly with a crush injury from a dropped object, students may think they only have a broken toe, but actually they've broken one or more metatarsals (long bones in the middle part of the foot). Additionally, tendon injuries can be more challenging than the fracture itself, creating drooping or flexed deformities of the finger or toe.

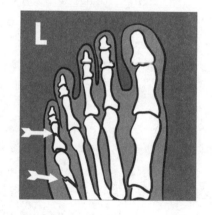

B. **Wrist fractures** come from falls—off scooters, bikes, stairs, curbs, and high heels. When you fall forward with an outstretched hand, the most commonly broken bones are the scaphoid (within your carpal wrist bones) and the radius, which is the larger of your forearm bones. The radius fracture typically occurs about an inch below the tip of your wrist, referred to as a "Colles" fracture. While these fractures are painful, often there is not dramatic swelling or bruising (and yes, you can still move all your fingers, though bending your wrist is uncomfortable). Not surprisingly, we often diagnose these fractures days or weeks after the injury.

C. **Stress fractures** are most common in the legs (tibia 23 percent, fibula 15 percent, femur 6 percent), feet (navicular 17 percent, metatarsal 16 percent), pelvis (1.6 percent), and spine (0.6 percent). Upper extremity stress fractures are rare, found in sports with overhead motions/throwing like pitching. The repetitive stresses cause microscopic fractures and disturb the normal bone remodeling process, causing more bone breakdown and not enough rest time to repair the damage.

Risk factors:
- **Running more than twenty-five miles per week**
- **Sudden increase in activity**
- Being female; especially with female athlete triad (eating disorders, thinning bones, and abnormal periods)
- Alcohol consumption of more than ten drinks per week
- Smoking
- Change in running surface or shoes

Stress fractures are often ignored or written off as a pulled muscle, shin splints, or "expected" soreness from a new workout program. These fractures often don't appear initially on X-rays, though they may be detected after a few weeks. If plain X-rays are negative but clinical suspicion is strong, your doctor may order an MRI or bone scan to better visualize the stress fracture.

Treatment:
Fracture treatment obviously is site- and injury-specific. Fortunately, the majority of fractures in college students can be managed with splinting, buddy taping, casts, walking boots, and braces, along with relative rest and rehab. Surgery may be required for displaced fractures to realign and possibly pin or screw the bones back in place.

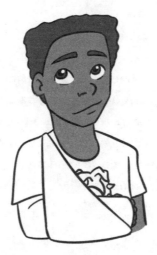

Rehab exercises are critical to return to full function and appearance.
- Take advantage of any physical therapy services provided by your university.
- Set reminders on your phone for daily exercises; they're boring but critical.

REST: Doctors hate diagnosing stress fractures because getting a runner to **stop running** is extremely difficult, and the *fracture will not heal until the same repetitive stress forces are removed.* Cycling and swimming are typically great alternate aerobic exercise choices, though clearly less convenient. Stress fractures take at least six to eight weeks to heal, requiring bracing, casting, or occasionally surgery.

Head to your doctor if:
- Your pain is severe and you lose feeling; or, if there is a visible deformity, seek immediate care.
- You have persistent pain, bruising, or swelling.
- Pain keeps you from normal activity with the affected area.

Worst-case scenario:

Initial worst case is requiring surgery, but the real worst case is missing or ignoring a fracture. Navicular fractures ache but rarely show bruising or swelling, and they are notoriously difficult to visualize on X-rays. Navicular bones are commonly injured by either a fall on outstretched hands (the wrist "navicular," a.k.a. scaphoid bone) or a stress/overuse injury in the foot. If these fractures are not recognized and properly treated, a combination of poor blood supply and failure to heal can result in long-term pain and disability.

Prevention:

- "Start low, go slow" when starting a workout or running program and be sure to cross-train. The majority of stress injuries come from overly aggressive single sport activity (usually running).
- Use your phone's flashlight. Better to briefly annoy/wake your roommates with a bit of light if you have to navigate the darkened room than to break your toe.
- Really try not to rush . . . allow at least an extra five minutes to get to classes or meetings. If you are a lifelong "late" person, NOW is the time to change that. Your future employers will appreciate the new "early" you.

TIPS:

- o **"I can move it, so it's definitely not broken" is a MYTH!** Movement comes from your ligaments, tendons, and muscles, and they can easily "move" a broken bone.
- o **Cross-train!** Physical therapy offices are filled with runners, not triathletes. Working the same muscle over and over will give you a stress injury.
- o New shoes: if you look at the tread on your shoes and see smooth areas from wear and tear, it's time for new running shoes.
  - o Old shoes are tough on feet/knees/hips; new shoes are cheaper than rehab.

○ Orthotics (custom-made or prefab like Powerstep or Spenco) can decrease the risk of stress injuries.

○ Toe fractures can often be treated with buddy taping and a hard-soled, inflexible (postop-type) shoe, but it's important to know what you're treating. X-rays often find more than one fracture. Especially if you are tender beyond your toe, see your doctor.

○ Shin splints make your shin tender to touch diffusely up and down the front of your leg, while a tibial stress fracture will be tender only in one discrete spot.

Chapter 48
Ankle Injuries, X-rays, and Expectations

What If: I Hurt My Ankle?
Medical Name: Ankle Sprain

What most likely happened:
College students have ample opportunities for twisting an ankle: intramural sports, rushing across campus and slipping in the rain or ice, stepping off of a curb "funny" or falling off high heels walking across an uneven parking lot. The typical injury is your foot buckling under to the inside (so the bottom of your injured foot is facing your other foot). The vast majority of all ankle injuries are sprains (85 percent), and then 85 percent of these sprains occur on the lateral (outside) ligaments.

What's going on?
When your foot buckles "inside," inverting the ankle, this stretches the outside of the ankle, and the weak spot that gives way first is the ligaments. The Anterior Talofibular Ligament (ATFL) is the most commonly injured ligament. If you touch the front part of your outside "ankle bone" and run your finger toward your toes about an inch, you will have an idea where this small ligament lives. The next most commonly injured ligament is

farther back, still on the outside/lateral part of your ankle, situated between your heel and the back of the bony tip of your ankle—the calcaneofibular ligament (CFL).

Do I need an X-ray?

Most sprains do NOT need an X-ray! Doctors use "Ottawa Ankle Rules" (which help accurately predict which acute injuries have a very low chance of including a broken bone) to decide whether to order an X-ray in order to reduce your radiation risk, time, and expense.

The Ottawa rules look at weight-bearing ability and tender spots on exam.

- Could you walk four steps right after your injury?
- Can you bear weight on your foot and walk four steps now?

If your answer is **yes** to both, an X-ray is likely not necessary (yet).

While examining you, your doctor will look for a few specific areas of tenderness to her touch, including the posterior, bony part of your ankle (both inner and outer) and then two spots on your foot where fractures are likely. If any one of these spots hurts worse when she presses directly on it, you'll be getting an X-ray to look for a broken bone.

Treatment:

Immediately after injury: RICE-PS

- **Rest**—Stop playing! Going back into a game after a mild injury is a great way to get a severe injury. For other situations, use relative rest. If bearing weight does not cause additional pain, take the shortest route to your next destination, catching a ride with a friend if possible.
- **Ice**—Ten minutes on, ten minutes off as much as you can for the first day or two. Avoid ice directly on the skin; frozen peas work great!
- **Compression**—Leave athletic shoe on until compression wrap is available (unless you are experiencing numbness, in which case you should remove the shoe).

- Elevation—Sit or lie down and prop up foot higher than your heart to minimize swelling.
- Pain relievers—Advil can ease pain and reduce swelling, Tylenol can help with pain.
- Splint—If you don't feel your injuries merit an immediate office visit, consider adding an OTC ankle splint (worn with shoes), either:
  - Hard plastic "stirrup"-style offers more support but is bulky.
  - Soft, less bulky lace-up with crisscrossing Velcro can be easier to wear with your sneakers.

Head directly to your doctor if:
- You can't bear weight on your foot.
- You have numbness, tingling, or weakness in your foot.
- You have excessive bruising or pain.
- Your symptoms are not steadily improving after several days.

Your clinician may add:
- **Prescription Ankle Brace, Splint, or Walking Boot**: These come in all shapes and sizes; work with your clinician to find one you will actually **wear** because this accessory should be your constant companion for the next six to eight weeks (*followed by use with every sport and significant weight-bearing activity for six to eight months*).
- **Crutches**: Goal generally is to get off crutches and bear weight as soon as possible, but severe sprains may require three to seven days of non-weight-bearing with crutches, followed by more time with crutches gradually adding weight bearing.
- **Temporary Parking Permit:** Do not **expect** this, but students with more severe injuries that require crutches may be given short-term parking permits to facilitate getting to class or work. Note that having a friend drop you off is often closer than designated parking!

Rehabilitation:

Reinjury after an ankle sprain is extremely common and can start a vicious cycle of "weak" ankle injuries. Therefore, the **most important part** of treating ankle sprains is focusing on regaining the lost flexibility, strength, and balance from the injury. *These exercises should be done every single day for at least six weeks.*

Foot flexion exercise: Seated and barefoot, and using your big toe, write the alphabet in both lower and upper case, not moving your leg (so only moving your toe, foot, and ankle).

Foot strength exercise: Still seated and barefoot, place a towel on the ground in front of you. Using only your toes, scrunch the towel, pulling it toward you one scrunch at a time till the whole towel has passed under your foot. Now place the towel sideways, and repeat using your toe scrunch and side-to-side motion to pull the towel left to right, using your toes, foot, and ankle, but not moving your leg.

Balance exercise: Stand on one leg, hands on your hips, for a timed one minute. Repeat on other leg. When you can easily do this, repeat the exercise with your eyes **closed.**

- **Pro tip:** Do this while you brush your teeth, one minute per foot, so you end up with both stronger ankles and healthier teeth and gums!

Worst-case scenario:

Your bad "sprain" turns out to be a broken bone, and in the very worst case, the broken bone(s) has separated and needs to be surgically repaired or pinned back in place.

Prevention:

- If you have any prior history of ankle injuries, do all three rehab exercises as part of your daily routine and wear ankle braces on both ankles for sports activities.

- High heel lover? Sorry, time to skip the stilettos and opt for wedges or flats.

TIPS:

○ Swelling and discomfort are **expected** for mild sprains, and their presence does not mean that you need an X-ray.

○ **Do not stop wearing your brace** after the pain goes away! For the next six to eight months, be sure to wear your brace for any significant exercise, sport, or activity.

○ If your ankle sprain isn't getting better, the **most common reason is that you are not faithfully doing all three daily rehab exercises** for a minimum of six weeks.

Chapter 49
Knee Pain without Injury (a.k.a. Too Many Stairs!)

What If: My Knee Hurts (without Any Injury)?

Medical Name: Patellofemoral Pain Syndrome

What most likely happened:

Halfway through fall semester, you started a running program to fend off the "Freshman Fifteen" weight gain, but now the front of your knee aches after sitting in class and hurts worse each time you climb up and especially when you go down stairs. It's hard to say exactly when it started, but the pain seems to be getting worse, and, at a minimum, the pain isn't going away. You never fell or twisted your knee, and frankly it looks perfectly normal—no obvious swelling or redness.

Should you go get an X-ray?

What's going on?

Patellofemoral Pain Syndrome (PFPS: patella = kneecap; femur = thigh bone) comes from a combination of overuse and muscle imbalance or weakness, rather than a one-time traumatic injury like a torn ligament or muscle strain. Women experience PFPS significantly more than men. Why? Because relatively broader hips create a wider "Q-angle" (quadriceps angle) at the knee, pulling the kneecap laterally and straining alignment. Running or jumping sports like basketball further increase that stress. In a healthy knee, cartilage serves as cushion between the kneecap and the leg bones. With PFPS, that cartilage is shredded or broken down (called *chondromalacia patella*), leaving the bones to basically grind against each other or at least against the now-jagged surface of the cartilage. Pain therefore worsens when you bear weight on a flexed knee, which explains why squatting or going up or down stairs hurts more than walking across campus.

Do you need an X-ray?

With no specific traumatic injury (no fall, car crash, sports collision, etc.) and a knee that looks normal but has pain behind the kneecap that is worse with squatting, **no**, an X-ray is not indicated yet! If, however, despite physical therapy and diligent home exercises for several weeks, you still have pain, some type of imaging may be considered.

Treatment:

The problems that cause PFPS are muscle imbalance, weakness, overuse, and abnormal kneecap tracking, so the mainstay of treatment is **exercise-based therapy**:

- **Strengthen the quadriceps**
- **Strengthen core trunk muscles**
- **Increase hamstring flexibility**

As with nearly all musculoskeletal problems, we also start with:

- **Relative rest**: Avoid stairs, squats, kneeling, and jumping but continue aerobic activities like walking, exercise biking against low resistance, or swimming.
- **Ice**: Ice pack to knees ten to twenty minutes after activity a few times per day
- **Ibuprofen or Naproxen**: As needed for pain relief short term (one week)

Do I need a knee brace?

Need? No, current evidence-based medicine says ***braces offer no benefit over exercise***, though in fairness, they also show no harm. Yes, there are braces designed to help with kneecap tracking and counteract the lateral pull of the quads, so if you want one, pick that style.

What about taping?

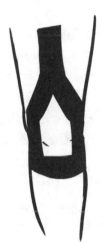

Maybe. If your pain started recently, properly taping the knee may transiently help reduce pain IF you also do physical therapy and exercise. ***Taping by itself*** *(without the rehab exercises)* ***does not help.*** Place the first piece of kinesiotape like an upside-down Y above and on either side of your kneecap, then secure that with a second piece of tape around your leg just below the kneecap. (Check with your PT or doctor to assure proper placement.)

Anything else?

Check your feet—specifically, look at the soles of your (athletic) shoes. **If the tread has worn off in sections, it's time for new shoes,** because this actually affects mechanical dynamics on your knees. Ladies, if you're routinely wearing heels and having knee pain, start with wearing flats (or better yet, if it's an option, go casual and wear sneakers). Additionally, although scientific studies are inconsistent, orthotic shoe inserts may also help with your knee pain, especially if you overpronate or have flat feet.

Head to your doctor if:

- You had an injury that started your knee pain.
- Your knee is visibly red or swollen.
- Your pain is increasing.
- Your knee is locking or giving way.

Worst-case scenario:

PFPS that does not respond to conservative treatment with physical therapy may ultimately require orthoscopic surgical intervention to smooth out the damaged cartilage. Interestingly, however, *the degree of visible cartilage breakdown does not directly correlate with the pain of this syndrome;* people may have much pain with little visible change or vice versa.

Prevention:

The best prevention is doing the same "treatment" exercises before you ever have pain, so again:
- **Strengthen the quadriceps.**
- **Increase hamstring flexibility.**
- **Strengthen core trunk muscles.**

Additionally:

"Start low, go slow" when beginning a new exercise program. Start a new running program with jogging one mile a few times per week, not jumping right into running three miles every day.

TIPS:

○ Patellofemoral pain can be in one or both knees, consistently felt as a deep ache in the front of the knee with occasional sharp pain (particularly when squatting or using stairs).

○ PFPS accounts for 30 to 40 percent of all doctor visits for knee pain and is one of the most common overuse injuries in running, volleyball, and basketball.

○ My favorite advice from sports medicine doctor Kristyn Fagerberg, MD, is "*There are no flip-flops with good arch support!* While you have knee, hip, or back pain, your feet belong in new athletic shoes—no flip-flops, and never walk barefoot."

○ Along with pain upon squatting or using stairs, PFPS can cause stiff and achy knees with prolonged sitting in a lecture (this is the so-called "theater sign"). Try sitting in an aisle seat where you can periodically extend and flex your legs during class.

KNEE EXERCISES (Prevention or Rehab of PFPS):
1. **Daily Straight Leg Lifts:**
    a. Sit up straight or lie flat on the floor with your "good" leg bent and "bad" leg straight with toes pointing straight up.
    b. Lift the "bad" leg about six to eight inches off the floor.
    c. Keep leg held steady while you slowly count to ten (one, Mississippi, two, Mississippi . . . ten).
    d. Lower leg and rest for five seconds.
    e. Repeat for a set of ten.
    f. Switch legs and do another set of ten on that leg.
    g. Finish the first part of exercise with a second set on each leg.
    h. Now keep your leg straight but rotate your foot outward about thirty degrees and repeat two sets of ten lifts per leg; you should feel this in your inner thigh (medial quad).

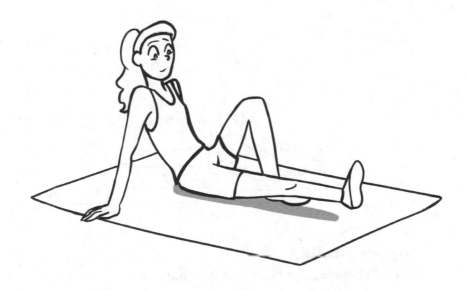

2. **Daily hamstring stretch**
   a. Lie flat with "good" leg straight and "bad" leg in the air, holding it with your hands on both sides of your thigh for support.
   b. Bend at the knee, flexing fully.
   c. Now extend as far as you can and hold for thirty seconds.
   d. Return to flexed/relaxed position and hold for five seconds, then repeat extension.
   e. Complete one set of five extensions, then switch legs and do the other side.
   f. Repeat both for a total of two sets per leg.

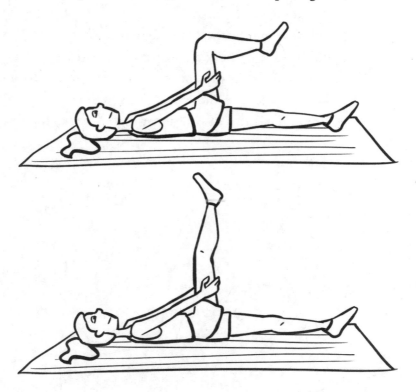

3. **Hip Strengthening**
   a. Stand balancing sideways on a bottom step, with your "good" leg on the step, and the "bad" leg off the step, hands

on your hips (grab the rail for support if you need it while you build up strength).

b. Keep your standing leg straight and slowly lower your other leg to toward the floor.

c. Using your gluteus muscles, now squeeze and raise your "floating" leg back up.

d. Repeat ten times, then change legs.

e. Goal: three sets of ten reps per leg.

4. **Classic Quad Sets**

a. Lie flat or sit against a wall with legs extended straight out, placing a rolled-up hand towel or small soft pillow underneath your knee.

b. Pull toes back toward your face while pushing down with your knee to flatten the towel/pillow.

c. Hold this pressure/contraction of your thigh muscle for about five seconds, then relax for several seconds.

d. Repeat ten times (on both legs).

e. **Classroom Modification**: While seated with your feet on the ground, simply tighten up your quad and hold for five seconds, then relax for several seconds and repeat. Goal is roughly ten reps per leg. Counting is not critical—the idea is to strengthen your muscles by squeezing in extra quad sets multiple times throughout the day while you are stuck in class or meetings.

Chapter 50
My Heel Hurts–
Especially That First Step!

What If: My Heel Hurts, Especially That First Step?
Medical Name: Plantar Fasciitis

What most likely happened:
Feeling motivated to get in shape, you signed up for your first 10K run and started training, ramping up your mileage as fast as possible. Although you never fell or injured your foot, now you've developed heel pain that is the absolute worst during the first few steps out of bed each morning. With more use, the pain dials down to a dull ache, but after sitting in class, the intense pain returns for the first several steps when you get up to head to your next class. Numbness, tingling, and burning that come from nerve compression are **not** part of this problem. Your most tender spot if you press on your heel is on the bottom, inner part.

What's going on?
Despite the commonly recognized "-itis" in plantar fasciitis, physicians now know that this is not problem of inflammation but one of degeneration. The thick band of tissue (called the plantar fascia) that runs on the

bottom of the foot develops microscopic tears as the collagen fibers that make up the fascia begin to break down.

Why did this happen?
- Tight heel cords: Present 70 percent of the time; you should be able to flex your foot back toward your face by fifteen degrees.
- Overaggressive training: trying to go too fast or too far too quickly
- Poor (overused or ill-fitted) shoes
- Flat feet **or** high arches
- Weak muscles in the foot

Treatment:
Symptomatic treatments include:
- Heel cups or heel donuts (pad with a cut-out center); place in your shoes and wear 24/7.
- Ice: ten-minute application to sore spot on heel a few times per day (frozen peas or a frozen plastic water bottle work great)
- Night splints (these stretch the heel cord all night)
- Physical therapy modalities with mild proven efficacy: phonophoresis or iontophoresis
- "Golf ball massage" using a golf ball, tennis ball, or other firm object to massage your foot; variations include freezing the ball first to combine ice and massage.

MOST IMPORTANT: Treatments that addresses the CAUSE:
- **Heel cord (Achilles) stretching**: Stand on stairs, holding rail, with one of your feet positioned halfway off stair and let your heel drop down till you feel the stretch in your calf; hold for thirty seconds, rest, and repeat several times. Repeat this set several times per day.
- **Training modification**: Only increase your distance by 10 percent per week, *but **first** cut back to **half** of previous training level before pain started.*

- **Check the bottom of your shoes**, and if you have areas of the tread that are worn smooth, it's time for new shoes!
- **Consider orthotics** to support high arches or flat feet
  - Start with OTC, but you may need custom-fitted orthotics.
  - If pain gets **worse** with orthotics, the orthotics are wrong—**stop**!
- **Foot-strengthening exercises**:
  - **Alphabet Writing**: Sitting down, cross-legged, write the alphabet with your big toe in upper then lower case.
  - **Towel Scrunch**: Place a towel flat on the floor in front of you, then using the toes of one foot, start grabbing the towel and pull it back toward you in progressive small scrunches, till you've eventually pulled the whole towel past your foot.

Head to your doctor if:
- Your pain is making you limp.
- You've tried the stretches, strengthening, ice, and cut back on your exercise but still hurt.
- You had a fall or other specific injury that started your pain.

Worst-case scenario:
Very rarely plantar fasciitis will persist beyond six to twelve months despite all these interventions, at which time you may require a physician-administered steroid heel injection or even surgery.

Prevention:
- Avoid overenthusiastic training too fast, too hard, too long.
- Invest in quality running shoes fitted by a trained salesperson (check local running shoe stores, or a local running club website for suggestions).

TIPS:

- **You do not need an X-ray for classic heel pain.**
- If you got an X-ray anyway, and there is a heel spur, **ignore it**; these spurs do not actually correlate with plantar fasciitis.
- Ibuprofen does **not** work well for this problem (beyond transient pain relief) because, remember, there is no inflammation.
- **Don't put new orthotics in old shoes.** *Got worn tread?* **Get new shoes!**

Chapter 51

I Stepped on a Nail (or Broken Glass)

What If: I Stepped on a Nail or Broken Glass?

Medical Name: Puncture Wound

What most likely happened:

Your high heels were killing your feet, so you're carrying them as you search the dimly lit parking lot for your car. Midtext, your foot suddenly erupts in pain—*what did you step on?* Parties and concerts are notorious for randomly scattered broken bottles and poking-up nails or splintered wood that can pierce your feet *even through thick sneakers*, but this happens most often to sandal-clad or bare feet.

Treatment:

- If possible, clean the wound by placing it under running water for several minutes and **wash, wash, wash!** More flushing = cleaner wound, better healing.
- Use liquid soap if handy, but do **not** scrub, and do **not** use peroxide, iodine, or alcohol. These products actually damage the skin and delay healing.

- If the nail or glass is not easily removed, or if you have fragments possibly still stuck in your foot, let your doctor remove it—**please do not dig around with your tweezers or a needle because** *this makes it harder for us and more uncomfortable for you;* our sterile equipment simplifies the process and avoids additional injury.
- X-ray or ultrasound may be necessary to look for fragments of glass or metal.
- Occasionally, we need to numb up your foot with local anesthetic to surgically remove the foreign object.

Head to your doctor if:

- These are "dirty" wounds—a risk for tetanus. If it's been **more than five years** since your last **tetanus** booster (your record will say Td or Tdap), then you need a booster now.
- **You stepped on a nail** *through your shoe*; this injury puts you at risk for a serious wound or bone infection from the bacterium *pseudomonas* (that often lives in sneaker soles), so you **need antibiotics**.
- You had a minor puncture wound a few days ago, but now there is increasing redness, swelling, pain, or fever.

Worst-case scenario:

- About 1.8 percent of puncture wounds will progress to infect a bone in your foot, which requires hospitalization and IV antibiotics.
- **Tetanus!** This easily preventable disease can be life-threatening.

Prevention:

- Keep your shoes on if you're outside.
- Use your phone's flashlight and **look** where you are walking, especially in fields and parking lots.

TIPS:

- **Keep the date of your last tetanus booster shot in your phone.**
- Avoid bare feet outside; resist the temptation to take painful shoes (yes, you, high heels!) off aching feet when walking back to your car/dorm/apartment.
- If you think you have something stuck in your foot, don't bear weight on that foot until it can be examined (seems obvious, but many people limp around on their foot and make it worse).
- Minor puncture wounds (like stepping on a tack or pin in your dorm room) can likely be treated at home if:
    - Your last tetanus shot was within five years.
    - You have no concern of fragments stuck in your foot.
    - Your puncture did not go through a shoe.

Cleanse thoroughly and use a topical antibiotic ointment; watch for signs of infection.

Chapter 52
Burns: A Matter of Degree

What If: I Got Burned?

Medical Name: First-, Second-, or Third-Degree Burns

What most likely happened:

Scenario A: Reaching back to grab your phone, you accidentally splash or knock over your mug of piping-hot coffee (or cheese slides off a pizza slice) onto your chest/arm/hand/leg.

Scenario B: Friday night, and your shared bathroom is overflowing with suitemates doing their makeup and hair. Though you're being careful not to burn your fingers with your curling wand, as you turn your head to respond to the roommate squeezing past you, the 400°F wand sears your forehead.

Scenario C: My e-cig or vape pen exploded!

What's going on?

In college health, most burns are thankfully minor injuries, often the result of rushing or distraction. What kind of burns do we see the most? Scalding burns from freshly microwaved liquids or foods and accidental encounters with stovetops, curling wands, or flat irons. Therefore, our primary concerns are to:

- Prevent secondary infection

- Promote healing to minimize scarring
- Ensure tetanus prophylaxis

Superficial first-degree burns are red, dry, and painful, only involving the epidermis.
- Typically heal within five to ten days
- Example: Classic sunburn without blisters

Superficial partial-thickness second-degree burns are red, wet, and painful, with clear weeping blisters that involve all the epidermis and the upper part of the underlying dermis.
- Typically heal within two weeks
- Usually don't scar
- Example: Sunburn with blisters

Deep partial-thickness second-degree burns still have the painful red, weeping blisters but also contain white areas.
- Take over three weeks to heal
- Frequently scar

Full-thickness third-degree burns become white-gray, tan, or brown, becoming numb and no longer painful because they extend through all skin layers and the underlying fat.
- Frequently require skin grafts
- Always scar

E-cigarette explosions are not common, but when they do occur, the burns are terrible. From 2015 to 2017, a total of 2,035 e-cig explosion burn injuries were reported from US hospital Emergency Rooms, and numbers continue to grow. The FEMA US Fire Administration report from 2017 showed that 31 percent of explosions occurred when the device or spare batteries were in a pocket, 31 percent occurred while it was being used, 25 percent while charging, and 9 percent while in storage. When these explosions occur in someone's mouth, hand, or pocket, there can obviously be extensive burn injuries.

Treatment:

Immediately:

- Remove any covering/clothing and nearby jewelry.
- Run cool water directly over the burn.
- Do **not** apply ice or immerse in ice water baths, as this *can cause further damage.*
- No need for cleaning agents beyond water; if you feel you need to use something, stick with a plain liquid soap (no alcohol, peroxide, etc., necessary, as they may further damage the tissue).
- Do **not** cover with butter, oils, or ointments (these substances retain heat and worsen the burn).
- Current vaccination guidelines from the ACIP recommend that if your last tetanus booster is more than five years ago and your burn is more than superficial (meaning blisters or worse), you need to get a **tetanus** booster shot.

Follow-Up Care:

- If desired, loosely cover burn with a sterile bandage.
- Superficial nonblistered first-degree burns: Clean once daily with a mild soap and water; you may use small amount of an OTC 1 percent hydrocortisone topical cream or a moisturizing lotion with aloe.
- OTC antibiotic products you may be used sparingly to prevent infection in partial-thickness burns.
- Blisters: Leave them alone; larger ones may be drained by a medical professional.
- Use oral OTC pain relievers as needed such as ibuprofen (preferred) and/or acetaminophen.
- Consider taking an OTC antihistamine such as Fexofenadine (Allegra), loratadine (Claritin), or cetirizine (Zyrtec) to limit the inflammatory response.
- More severe burns may require prescription dressings and antibiotics (topical or oral).

Head to your doctor if your burn is:

- On your face, fingers, toes, genitals, or over a joint (meaning knees, not pot!).
- Large (greater than two to three inches), deep (any blisters), or intensely painful.
- All the way around the body section (finger/arm, etc.).
- Looking infected—expanding redness beyond the initial burn— or if you develop a fever.

Worst-case scenario:

Typical worst case for minor college student burns is secondary infection (usually from scratching or picking at healing wounds) and scarring.

Severe burns—including inhalation, chemical, electrical, and any type of burn that covers more than 10 percent of your body or is located on your face, hands, feet, genitals, or covering large joints—should be treated at a specialized burn center.

Prevention:

- Microwaves are often added to tight spaces; be sure to place your microwave below eye level, because reaching up makes you more likely to spill.
- Cook on the back burners if multiple people are around.
- Curling wands: Use the gloves provided and curl front sections **away** from your face.
- Place a floating shelf in the bathroom for phone storage while doing hair and makeup.
- Unplug irons from the wall—do not leave hot irons near edges of tables or counters.
- Wear hats, use sunscreen, and do **not** use tanning beds.

TIPS:

- Sunscreen: Apply a shot-glass size of lotion to your body every two hours for full protection.
- The **worst sunburns** come from:

o Not realizing your antibiotic or acne medication makes you
   photosensitive
   o Tetracycline medications: doxycycline and
      minocycline
   o Trimethoprim sulfamethoxazole (Bactrim)
o Falling asleep (or passing
   out from alcohol) while
   sunbathing/partying
   outside
o Not using sunscreen
   because it's cloudy out
o High-altitude sports (snow
   skiing)
o All-day outdoor spectator
   sporting events (tailgates
   and games)

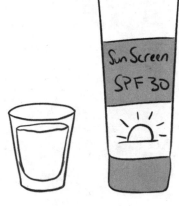

o Getting a "base tan" does not
   prevent sunburns (skip the tanning salon before Spring Break!).
o Your last tetanus shot was likely seventh grade (unless you've had
   reason to get another); if your burn has blisters, your doctor will
   likely recommend a booster shot.

Chapter 53
Acne, "Backne," and Cysts

What If: I Get Acne, "Backne," or Cysts?
Medical Name: Acne vulgaris, Pilonidal Cyst

What most likely happened:
Scenario A: In high school, you had your share of annoying pimples, enough that your doctor prescribed a cream to use with flare-ups. That prescription has expired, and now not only is your face breaking out, but so is your chest and back. You've tried scrubbing your hardest with Buf-Pufs, special soaps, and every extra-strength acne product with no success.

   Scenario B: You recently started on birth control pills to improve your painful periods, and now your face is completely broken out. The women's health providers keep telling you that you need to give it more time, but you don't want to spend the whole semester in the zit zone.

   Scenario C: Your acne has been reasonably well controlled, but now somehow you have this huge, tender red bump near the top of your butt crack that looks like a giant, swollen, painful pimple.

What's going on?
Scenarios A and B: Acne plagues the majority of adolescents and young adults at one point or another, and no one solution is foolproof, which is obvious if you look at the vast array of OTC acne products. Multiple

factors are involved, starting with hormonally increased oil production and clogged follicles, then bacteria (*Propionibacterium acnes*) set up shop, and all this activity triggers an inflammatory reaction. Noninflammatory blackheads or whiteheads created by partially or fully clogged follicles may progress to pimples and painfully inflamed cystic nodules.

Do birth control pill hormones cause acne? Yes and no. The "minipill," which only contains progesterone (and no estrogen), can definitely cause acne. However, combination estrogen/progesterone birth control pills can be extremely effective in treating acne, particularly in women who experience acne flares the week before their period. While other brands may also help, only three pills are officially FDA-approved for acne treatment: *Estrostep, Ortho Tri-Cyclen,* and *Yaz.* Each of these pills contains a unique type of progesterone, with different indications and side effects that your doctor will consider as she chooses which best fits with your complete medical history. However, none of these pills is consistently superior to the others for acne treatment, and acne flare-ups are not uncommon the first month or two when starting a new pill. There are obviously many variables involved with acne, but even if your skin was totally clear before starting the pill and now suddenly you are breaking out, the first step is probably going to be maximizing topical skin treatments with benzoyl peroxide and topical antibiotics rather than immediately switching pills. Yes, sometimes we do need to switch pills, even before three months (which is our standard trial period for a new birth control pill), but unfortunately acne response is typically timed in months, not days.

Scenario C: This painful bump is NOT a pimple, but a *pilonidal cyst* (pilus = hair; nidus = nest). Although these are not common in the general population, we see these routinely in college students. Why? Because they occur most commonly in young adults—Caucasian males in particular, though not exclusively. A mixture of genetic predisposition, friction from prolonged sitting, hormones, and coarse or excess hair combine to create a cyst that surrounds what may have started as an ingrown hair. Ultimately these cysts become infected, which means you develop a painful, enlarging red bump, with bonus foul-smelling discharge.

Treatment:

Acne:

- **Benzoyl peroxide:** Topical products (gel, foam, lotion, creams, and cleansers) work to dry up the skin and reduce the bacteria that cause acne; they are especially effective when combined with prescription topical or oral antibiotics.
- Benzoyl peroxide washes (like Panoxyl) are EXCELLENT for facial and body acne. Leave on for a full five minutes before washing off, and use white towels or expect to find white blotches on your towels because the benzoyl peroxide will absolutely bleach them as you dry off.
- **Salicylic acid:** Topical products (disposable pads to creams, cleansers, lotions or sprays) focus on unclogging follicles and getting rid of the excess dead skin cells.
- **Azelaic acid** (prescription brands Azelex and Finacea): topical cream, foam, or gel with some antibacterial and anti-inflammatory properties; works better combined with erythromycin.
- **Antibiotics:**
  - Topical clindamycin can reduce the redness and inflammation by killing your acne-causing bacteria. This product is especially effective when combined with benzoyl peroxide, which helps prevent the development of antibiotic resistance.
  - Dapsone is a topical anti-inflammatory gel that may be tried if clindamycin is not tolerated. However, this can NOT be used along with benzoyl peroxide, because that combination causes a transient (up to two months) yellow-orange discoloration of the skin and facial hair.
  - Oral antibiotics may be used daily for an extended period (several months or more) for more severe acne. The most commonly prescribed antibiotics are tetracycline (doxycycline or minocycline) and trimethoprim/

sulfamethoxazole. Although they are generally well tolerated, the most common associated side effects for these medications are upset stomach (nausea or diarrhea) and photosensitivity (adverse skin reactions to sunlight).

- **Topical retinoids** (Differin, Tazorac, Retin-A): Prevent blackhead and whitehead formation, so these medications can be prescribed as single therapy for mild, noninflammatory acne. For more severe inflammatory acne (with pustules, cysts, and nodules), these topical agents can be combined with antibiotics.

- **Oral retinoids:** Isotretinoin (most recognized brand name Accutane) is reserved to treat severe, nodular, or cystic acne that did not improve with all other acne medications. Isotretinoin works by dramatically decreasing skin oil (sebum) production. Expected side effects may include sensitive, dry skin; cracked lips; and/or dry eyes. Other conditions that have been associated with isotretinoin include depression, muscle pains, and pancreatitis. The most serious potential side effect, however, is the possibility of severe birth defects if you were to get pregnant while taking this drug. Isotretinoin is an extremely effective medication, but because of the potentially severe side effects, physicians, patients, and pharmacists must all adhere to the mandated iPledge program requirements to ensure female patients will not conceive while taking this drug.

- **Oral contraceptives:** Estrostep, Ortho Tri-Cyclen, and Yaz are the FDA-approved pills to treat acne in females. These medications decrease the amount of skin oil production by lowering the levels of androgen hormones in your body. (Androgens are often called "male" hormones because they include testosterone, but these hormones are present in both genders.)

- **Spironolactone:** This medication also decreases skin oil production, but rather than lowering androgen levels, it works by blocking the effects of androgens directly on the glands that produce skin oil. The American Academy of Dermatology notes that spironolactone works best in women with acne along their jawline and lower face. Overall, evidence is still conflicting on this medication's efficacy, but spironolactone remains an option for females with hormonally aggravated, treatment-resistant acne.

Pilonidal cyst:
Antibiotics are not the answer for an infected cyst; the critical initial treatment is a minor surgical procedure. Your doctor will numb the skin with a shot of local anesthetic, then make a small incision to drain the cyst. *Does this hurt?* Yes, it's an uncomfortable brief procedure, but patients say the relief they feel once the pressure is released is more than worth it. Do *not* suffer in silence thinking this will clear up on its own, because typically these merely smolder and get worse. Unfortunately, these cysts are often complex, extending far deeper than you might expect, so recurrence is common after a simple drainage procedure. For complete, definitive removal of the cyst, you will need a surgical referral to a specialist.

Head to your doctor if:
- Your acne is upsetting or embarrassing you.
- You've tried a consistent OTC hygiene regimen for a month and your acne is worse.
- You're using prescription topical medications without improvement for six to eight weeks.
- You see a clear pattern of acne breakouts related to your menstrual cycle.
- You have a painful bump down near the cleft in your buttocks (don't wait for it to get "bad" enough that you cannot sit or lie down!).

Worst-case scenario:
Scarring is typically the worst case for acne, both physically and emotionally. On the physical side, acne may leave skin darkened or lightened (hyper- or hypopigmentation), indented or puckered with "pock" marks, or raised with overreactive "keloid" scars. Physicians can offer many treatment options from simple topical prescription bleaching agents to more invasive

procedures like chemical peels, dermabrasion, collagen or fat injections, and laser skin resurfacing.

Emotional scarring from acne is perhaps more difficult to treat. Particularly with severe acne, self-image can plummet and trigger depression, anxiety, and social withdrawal. *If your acne—regardless of the severity—is negatively affecting how you interact with others at school or socially, please make an appointment to see your doctor.* Acne treatments are not overnight solutions, so we want to get started treating you as early as possible!

Prevention:

- **Hygiene:** Acne does not mean you have poor hygiene, because hormones, genetics, medications, environment, etc., all affect your skin, most of which you cannot control. Maximizing your skin hygiene, however, is something that you can control:
  - Wash your face twice daily using a mild cleanser, water, and your hands (no "scrubber" like Buf-Pufs, powered face-scrubbers, or wash cloths) and rinse well, then gently pat dry with a clean towel.
  - Dermatologists strongly recommend NOT using makeup wipes to remove makeup, but instead, do a double cleanse with either micellar water or an oil cleanser, followed by a gentle soap (like Cerave Foaming Facial Cleanser).
  - If your skin becomes dry (which often happens if you are using acne products), use a small amount of acne-friendly oil-free moisturizing lotion like Neutrogena Facial Moisturizer or consider combination moisturizer and sunscreen products such as Cetaphil Pro Oil Absorbing Moisturizer SPF 30 or CeraVe AM.
  - **Sunscreen:** The best way to protect your skin's health and minimize discoloration from acne scarring is consistent use of sun protection including wearing hats and applying daily sunscreen. If your moisturizer didn't contain any SPF, add a thin layer of "noncomedogenic" sunscreen.

- **Makeup:** Be sure to choose "noncomedogenic" and oil-free products, and if you use a base, consider one that contains salicylic acid such as Neutrogena's Skin-Clearing Oil-free Makeup or Clinique Acne Solutions Makeup.

- **Diet:** Conventional wisdom says you should give up dairy and chocolate, but does science support that? Maybe not—current evidence primarily blames high glycemic load diets for acne exacerbations. High glycemic index foods break down quickly into simple sugars, so classic examples are "complex carbs" like chips, pastas, refined breads, cookies, and cereals. Dairy has been only weakly associated with acne flares. If you want to see if dairy-free makes a difference for your skin, please be sure that you are getting enough calcium in your diet. And chocolate? The jury is still out. It's not unhealthy to give up chocolate, so if you see a difference in your skin that makes it worthwhile, do it. My advice is to fill your diet with veggies, fruits, and protein, drink more water than anything else, and simply enjoy sweets like chocolate and high glycemic foods like pasta in moderation.

- **Hair Products:** Remember that everything you put in your hair basically ends up on your facial skin (either directly or courtesy of your pillow at night), so oil-based shampoos and alcohol-based hair sprays can aggravate your face and body acne. Consider an oil-free or antiresidue shampoo like Neutrogena antiresidue shampoo and remember to use your body scrub/soap **after** you finish your hair, so you can be sure you've cleaned the hair products off your skin.

- **Shower asap after workouts:** Working up a sweat is awesome for your heart, but not so great for your skin if you don't cleanse as soon as possible. Especially in a dorm room, where your bed is all you've got, shower **before** you kick back and relax. Seriously, avoid the postworkout temptation to collapse on your bed while checking social media or playing video games.

TIPS:

○ **Wash your sheets more often:** the goal is weekly, but at least shoot for twice a month and change your pillow cases twice a week (easy to have extra pillow cases—not much to store, and it doesn't add much to your hamper, but it can make a big difference with your acne).

○ **Get rid of the scrubbers** like Buf-Pufs and powered face-scrubbing brushes and use only your hands, water, and acne cleanser/soap to gently but thoroughly wash your face.

    ○ *Overly aggressive scrubbing makes acne worse.*

○ **Buying OTC benzoyl peroxide plus a prescription antibiotic cream** is often less expensive than purchasing the prescription combined antibiotic/benzoyl peroxide product; talk to your doctor and pharmacist to determine the most cost-effective method with your health insurance.

○ Back acne often responds very well to a combination of benzoyl peroxide wash (like Panoxyl) and a salicylic acid spray. Be sure to LEAVE ON the benzoyl peroxide wash for about five minutes before rinsing or it won't be very effective!

○ Bonus tip: For excellent body and foot odor control: use generous amounts of benzoyl peroxide wash in your armpits and on your feet (again, leave on for five minutes before washing off).

○ **Doxycycline** (or minocycline) is best absorbed on an empty stomach, but if that makes you nauseated, try taking your pill with a dense nondairy snack (like a high-protein granola bar).

○ Never hesitate to talk with your primary care physician or a dermatologist about your acne! There are many prescription medications that can help and you may need assistance choosing which OTC products are best for your skin.

Chapter 54
Bites, Stings, and Blistering Things

What If: Something STUNG or BIT Me?

Medical Names: Insect Sting or Bite; Herpes Simplex Virus; Contact Dermatitis

What most likely happened:

You're unlikely to miss the sudden sharp sting of a bee, wasp, or hornet, and you probably know to immediately apply an ice pack and possibly take an antihistamine (Benadryl) if the redness, swelling, or pain increase. But what if that sting is from a *scorpion*? Or if you unwittingly step ankle-deep into a fire ant mound at the edge of a lake while climbing into a boat? Or you discover a tick on your arm after camping and are freaking out about Lyme disease? And what's that itchy pimple-looking thing on your leg . . . could it be a poisonous black widow or brown recluse spider bite? Dr. Google suggests you might die!

What's going on?

Every part of the country has unique pests, so if you are in college far from home, don't wait for a sting or bite to learn about the risky insects in your new location.

Students tend to come in:

1. Immediately after a sting because of lip swelling, trouble swallowing or breathing, chest tightness, flushing, and/or nausea due to a severe allergic anaphylactic reaction—*this is a true emergency!*
2. Immediately after exposure because they are **terrified** that any scorpion sting or spider bite is extremely toxic, and they're not sure how to treat it.
3. When they notice a single pustule or a cluster of "bites" on their body that they assume is a spider bite, although have no memory of feeling or seeing an insect (this may actually be an infection or contact dermatitis, not a bite/sting).
4. When they have bites or stings "too numerous to count" usually on the feet and ankles (fire ants or fleas).

Treatment:

- Initial treatment for all insect bites or stings* is to wash area with soap and water, then apply a cold compress (ice pack), followed by topical steroid (OTC hydrocortisone) cream and/or oral antihistamine (Allegra, Claritin, or Zyrtec) are first choices; the older first generation, diphenhydramine/Benadryl, is now a second choice), if needed.
  - *If stinger is stuck in your skin, use fingernails or an ID card to scrape over the stinger and flick it away; avoid using tweezers because that forces more venom into your skin.
- If you have a known severe allergy to that insect and have an Epi-Pen, use it at the first sign of symptoms: swelling, hives, flushing, nausea, abdominal cramps, shortness of breath, cough, racing heart, metallic taste, itchy throat, or trouble swallowing—do NOT wait for symptoms to become severe. If you use the Epi-Pen, follow your doctor's directions for the next step (don't assume you are "one and done").

- Your doctor may prescribe oral steroids if oral antihistamines and topical steroids aren't helping enough, especially if you have excessive numbers of bites/stings.
- Antibiotics are typically only needed when you aggressively scratch your itchy bites and end up with a secondary bacterial skin infection (cellulitis).
- If you live in the Northeast or Midwest **and** you had a tick attached to you for more than thirty-six hours **and** you saw your doctor within three days of the tick bite, she may choose to give you a single dose of antibiotics to prevent the development of Lyme disease.

Head to your doctor if:
- You have any shortness of breath, trouble swallowing, lip swelling, chest tightness, abdominal pain or nausea, or dramatically increasing swelling or redness around your bite/sting.
- Your bite "bump" turns into an open sore, or you develop fever or progressively increasing redness, tenderness, or swelling around the bite/sting.
- You develop a rash (especially a bull's-eye rash after a tick bite), joint pain, or fevers.

Worst-case scenario:
Anaphylaxis: A severe multisystem allergic reaction that typically starts within five to thirty minutes after the bite/sting, which, **if left untreated**, can lead to shock and even death.

- **Bad news**: *Young, healthy people often underestimate the serious nature of warning signs.*
- **Good news**: Knowing these **warning signs** allows you to seek help quickly, which means someone administering an EpiPen (if available) can call 911 if the sting/bite victim develops any:
  - Flushing or hives
  - Trouble breathing or swallowing
  - Swollen lips
  - Nausea, vomiting, diarrhea, or abdominal cramps
  - Feeling faint or passing out

Prevention:

Cover Your Skin: If you are going to work cleaning out storage, go hiking in the woods, or hang out in any place infrequently visited by humans, use hats, work gloves, closed-toe shoes, and long pants and long-sleeve shirts.

Fire Ants: *SEC schools, I'm talking to you!* These pests are primarily in the southeastern United States. Locals know not to run barefoot in the grass or next to sidewalks or edges of lakes, especially after a soaking rain (that causes ant mounds to seek dryer ground). Main prevention is wearing shoes and looking at the ground as you walk.

Bee/Hornet/Wasp Stings: Don't look or smell like a flower if you're hanging around outside (seriously—no brightly colored shirts or floral perfumes).

Spiders and Scorpions: Especially if you live in the Southwest, wear shoes to walk around at night and shake out shoes and clothing before you put them on if you are picking them up off the floor. Especially at dusk, beware picking up blankets, boxes, patio furniture covers, etc., where these insects may have scurried in to spend the day hiding in the shade.

TIPS:

- **Fire ants** will aggressively swarm (especially when you accidentally step into a mound) and will likely be all over your legs when suddenly they all seem to sting at once. Do NOT spray them with water or shake your legs to remove them, because that will simply trigger them to sting more and cling tighter. Best removal method is fast, repetitive brushing off.

○ **Tick** removal should be done with **tweezers** (versus never use tweezers for stray bee stingers). Do **not** waste time trying to burn them with a match or smothering them with Vaseline or nail polish, just grab the tick right at your skin and pull straight up.

○ **Lyme Disease** comes from deer ticks in grassy, wooded areas in the Northeast and Midwest; if you remove the tick from your skin within a day, your risk of contracting Lyme disease is extremely low, so **cover up** while outdoors and **look closely** at your body each night.

○ **Brown recluse spiders** live in the Midwest and South-Central United States, typically shy and hiding in dark, warm, dry spots like under rocks, woodpiles, boxes, or corners of storage units. This spider ranges in size from a nickel to a quarter with its skinny, smooth light-brown legs extended and have a violin shape on top up near the head. People typically discover the bite many hours after it happened, starting with an itchy red bump that may blister, then become an open sore. Although *the vast majority of bites from this spider will resolve without medical intervention*, about 10 percent can become severe and require antibiotics to avoid a gangrenous response. Keep in mind these are not common even within their geographic area, and virtually unheard of in other parts of the United States.

○ **Scorpion** bottom line: outside of Arizona and portions of southern California and Utah (where the dangerous Bark Scorpion resides), consider scorpion stings to be extra painful bee stings—burning and hurting like crazy initially, but local ice pack application and OTC pain control (studies usually recommend aspirin over others) should be all you need. *If you do live in the Bark Scorpion zone,* then know that signs of more severe scorpion envenomation, which would require immediate medical care, include shortness of breath, increasing area of numbness, muscle twitching, or seizures. For the Bark Scorpion, antivenom may be required (only used about one hundred times each year, mostly for the very young or old).

o **Black Widow spider bites** typically occur when you accidentally sit on (think outhouse) or touch one while blindly grabbing something that the spider is sitting on, like a stick from a woodpile. Recognize this shiny black, nickel-to-quarter-sized spider by the red hourglass on its bottom.

o **Snap a pic** on your phone rather than trying to capture the insect if you actually see your perpetrator.

o **Epi-Pen Injection:** "Blue to the sky, Orange to the thigh." Hold the pen along the barrel (don't touch top or bottom), pull the blue cap straight off, then jab (and hold) the orange end into the upper outer thigh, through clothes if leg is not exposed, and hold for a count of five. Then call 911—*do not assume you're fully cured.*

o Know when campus doctors see your complaint is "spider bite" on your buttocks or upper leg, what we are **expecting** to see is actually genital herpes (most commonly obtained from receiving oral sex). **STDs are COMMON; bad spider bites are RARE.**

  o See Chapter 45: Sexually Transmitted Infections (Yes, It Happens to People like You) starting on page 221.

o Some "bites"—itchy red bumps or blisters—are not actually bites, but **contact dermatitis** like **Poison Ivy, Poison Oak, and Poison Sumac.**

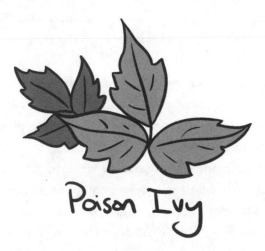

Poison Ivy

Key points about poison ivy:
- About 60 to 80 percent of the population will react to **urushiol**, the plant's poison sap.
- Urushiol can be spread by directly touching the root, stem, or leaf of these plants and by clothing or animal fur. If you and your dog romped through the brush, she might be part of your exposure, so use rubber gloves to shampoo her to remove the urushiol and add the leash to your next load of wash. *Human-to-human contact from the rash does NOT spread this dermatitis.*
- *NEVER* burn these plants—the inhaled smoke can damage your nose, throat, and lungs with a severe allergic reaction.
- **How soon do you break out?** Depends how many times you have previously been exposed. The first time, you may have a gap of several days before you start itching, but each successive breakout will occur *more quickly* and often will be *more severe*. Previously sensitized people may begin itching within minutes to hours of contact. Severe reactions can progress to full anaphylaxis with symptoms including shortness of breath, swollen lips (or swollen tongue or throat), nausea, vomiting, a racing or weak pulse, and sudden low blood pressure (which can make you pass out).
- Red bumps are often in a line (from the leaf swiping your leg), but if spread by pet fur or material, you may have patches, as well.
- Bumps become blisters that ooze clear fluid when scratched.
- Scratching can cause a secondary bacterial skin infection that may require antibiotics.
- **Heat makes the itch worse**; take cool showers and use ice packs.
- OTC oral antihistamines and topical steroid (hydrocortisone) creams work for mild cases, but severe rashes typically require prescription oral steroids.
- Head to the doctor if you have any wheezing/shortness of breath, any rash on or near your genitals or on your face, rash that extends beyond one extremity, or a possible skin infection (redness, swelling, discolored drainage or fever).

Chapter 55

Skier's Toe: Campus Version (Painful, Black Toenail or Fingernail)

What If: My Toenail or Fingernail Is Black and Painful?

Medical Name: Subungual hematoma (Bleeding beneath the nail)

What most likely happened:

Scenario A: After an awesome day of downhill skiing (or hiking in new boots, playing soccer or tennis), you take off your boots only to discover your big toe toenail is half blackened and super painful to touch.

Scenario B: Mover's remorse: Someone (possibly you) dropped a heavy box of books or dorm furniture on your toes or fingers (perhaps attempting to insert bed risers or maneuvering a desk under your lofted bed) or you accidentally hit your finger with a hammer or caught a finger in a door.

What's going on?

Repetitive jamming of toes against a stiff box or direct trauma to a toe or fingernail both result in bleeding underneath the nail. The problem is that this blood has nowhere to go because it is trapped between the nail bed and the nail itself, so even a few drops of blood create tremendous pressure and throbbing pain. The nail may first look bluish purple but quickly turns black.

Treatment:

Very small under-the-nail bleeds may be tolerable and can be treated symptomatically with ice, elevation, and time. However, the only way to relieve rapidly increasing pressure and pain is to directly remove the blood by creating a small hole (or series of several holes) in the nail.

Please do not try this at home!

Dr. Google may suggest saving the expense of a doctor's visit by trying to perform this minor surgery using a flame-sterilized hot paper clip to burn the hole, and while that is one technique that can be used, be forewarned: **this toenail surgery is famous for making people pass out**. The combination of intense pain plus seeing blood ooze up through the holes is powerful. Seriously. Don't trade your throbbing toe for a head injury from fainting. Your clinician most likely has an electrocautery tool (or at least sterile needles) and the clinical expertise and experience to very quickly penetrate the nail and release the blood, typically providing relief in a matter of seconds. Remember that nails, like hair, feel no pain (think about haircuts), so understand the pain involved in this procedure is only the brief extra pressure on your already throbbing toe. In contrast, inexperienced, nervous hands can drag this out and potentially cause damage by going in too far—enough said.

Head to your doctor:

The sooner, the better! If you wait a day or two, the blood will likely become clotted and therefore not drain easily, which means you may go through the procedure but get minimal relief. If your pain is merely a nuisance, wait it out, but if you wince when you touch your nail, go get it fixed.

Worst-case scenario:

When these nail bleeds happen from a direct blow like a car door or hammer, the fingertip bone underneath may be cracked or "broken," so X-rays may be needed in addition to draining the nail. Additionally, the nail bed blood vessels may not only be smashed, but actually torn, in which case they must be repaired by stitching them closed. This injury is suspected when the nail discoloration covers more than half of the nail and most commonly occurs when the nail is already visibly deformed (cut across or coming off). Obviously, to suture the blood vessels, the nail will need to be at least partially removed to allow the clinician access for suturing. Rest assured, we do use local anesthesia before these more involved interventions.

Prevention:

Properly fitted athletic shoes and ski boots are a must. Ski boots are particularly challenging because, frankly, they are nearly all uncomfortable. The key is that your foot should not be able to slide forward, so the problem comes more often from people thinking they need "looser" boots than from ones that feel too tight.

Wear closed-toed shoes when moving in and out of dorms; cute sandals and flip-flops offer zero protection.

TIPS:

- *Will your nail fall off after being drained?* Depends on the size of your bleed. Often the nail will remain intact, in which case you will see the discolored area slowly and steadily advancing as it grows out to the end of the nail. Fingernails take three to six months to grow back, while toenails take much longer—a year to eighteen months.
- Other more serious medical problems (like melanoma skin cancer) can very rarely cause darkening of your nails, so if you don't remember any obvious injury to your finger or toenail, do not ignore it—get it checked out!

Chapter 56
Piercing Problems

What If: I'm Having "Piercing" Problems?

Medical Names: Stuck Foreign Body, Laceration, Cellulitis, or Allergic Dermatitis

What most likely happened:

Scenario A: You suddenly realize the back of your earring is gone . . . *and it must be stuck inside your earlobe* because you can't pull the earring out from the front, and the back of the ear may even appear to be closed off.

Scenario B: Rushing to change clothes, you pull your sweater off over your head only to have the knit loops snag your earring, and the subsequent tug-of-war leaves you with a torn, bleeding ear lobe.

Scenario C: The immediate area around your piercing is red, itchy, painful, and possibly oozing. Is this infection or allergy?

What's going on?

A: Overly tight earring clasps or local irritation (with or without infection) can encourage stud earrings to migrate forward and get "sucked inside" your ear. Initially the hole remains open, but if ignored, with time the skin will grow over and fully embed the back half of your earring within your ear. The discomfort ranges from annoyance to sleep disrupting, depending on the degree of infection.

B: Torn earlobes are painfully common, especially with larger, hooped earrings that provide an easy target for flailing fingers in tightly packed, exuberant sporting events or on crowded dance floors. Equally common, however, are the self-induced rips from accidental hair or clothing snags, which can happen with any style of earring.

C: Ears, belly-button, and nose piercings commonly develop redness, itching, and pain, and the challenge is determining whether this is local irritation from an allergic reaction to metal (most commonly nickel) or you've developed a skin infection. Note that even pure gold earrings are often paired with posts or backs that contain blends of metal with nickel and white gold almost always contains nickel, unless it is specified to be palladium white gold. Pain, discolored discharge, expanding redness, and significant swelling suggest infection versus the discomfort, intense itch, primarily hole-focused redness, and clear discharge or scaly skin of allergic reactions. However, symptoms often overlap, especially with fresh piercings, which are effectively open wounds.

Treatment:

A: For stuck earrings, **please go in** and let a doctor remove or repair it as soon as possible. *I'm serious—put down those tweezers!* Messing around and attempting to fix these problems yourself usually cause much more pain, lead to worse infections, and complicate the removal procedures. We can numb up the area with local anesthetic (topical cream and/or a small injection) and use sterile instruments to access and typically retrieve your earring within a few minutes. Topical antibiotics are usually enough to treat infection in the ear lobe, but if your piercing was stuck in the cartilage, you likely need oral antibiotics. Cartilage has no direct blood supply because it contains no blood vessels, making it difficult for antibiotics to reach the infection. Additionally, the ear cartilage infections are often caused by a resistant bacterium (Pseudomonas) that is not affected by our usual first-choice antibiotics.

B: Torn earlobes often require referral to a plastic surgeon, dermatologist, or ENT surgeon. Ripped earlobes may not bleed too much, given their poor blood supply. Use gauze to hold pressure and stop the bleeding, and head to an urgent care or ER to be treated. Do not apply ice directly to the skin, but you may use a cool compress if desired to help with pain control. Do **not** try to use superglue—this doesn't work in inexperienced hands because you can't properly line up the edges, and the end result is a distorted shape. Additionally, glue can seal in bacteria (leading to an abscess), and subsequently, all of this makes the surgeon's job more difficult. This repair is a minor surgery done in the office with local anesthesia and precise, tiny stitches for the best cosmetic outcome.

C: For irritated, red, and itchy established piercings, remove the jewelry and cleanse area twice daily with generously saline solution–soaked gauze, followed by OTC hydrocortisone cream. If the redness expands beyond a couple millimeters, or you develop pain, swelling, or pus, head in to your doctor. New piercings often ooze clear to light-yellow discharge as they are healing. Therefore, if you are not having significant pain or swelling, try treating irritated new piercings by leaving in the jewelry and simply cleansing with the saline-soaked gauze twice daily. Some clinicians recommend trying OTC antibiotic preparations for noncartilage infections, but if you try that and your irritation gets worse, you may be having an allergic reaction to the neomycin component. Neomycin is the most common topical antibiotic to cause a contact allergy, with an estimated prevalence of 1 to 9 percent. Doctors often avoid neomycin for this reason, prescribing a different antibiotic like mupirocin (Bactroban) instead.

Head to your doctor if:
- You realize all or part of your piercing has become embedded inside your ear/nose/cartilage, etc.
- You have **any cartilage piercing** that looks or feels infected (increasing redness and tenderness—don't wait for pus and fever).
- You think you are allergic to your piercing jewelry, but symptoms persist after removal plus several days of home treatment with saline cleansing and OTC hydrocortisone cream.

Worst-case scenario:
Serious infections from piercings may progress enough to require hospitalization and IV antibiotics, primarily in the case of **cartilage** piercing

infections. More commonly, however, the worst case is a poor cosmetic result from scarring after an infection or a traumatic tear (from a yanked piercing).

Prevention:

- To avoid embedded earrings, use larger back clasps and do not overly tighten, or choose loop-style earrings that do not require clasps.
- Remove earrings before you sleep and clean them weekly with alcohol or sanitizer to remove the shampoo, hair products, and dead skin cells that naturally build up and collect on the jewelry.
- Remove earrings before playing sports or caring for babies and toddlers. (Dangling earrings are **irresistible**!)

TIPS:

- About 20 percent of earlobe piercings (*versus 30 percent of cartilage piercings*) become infected even with conscientious hygiene. While earlobe infections are easily treated, cartilage infections are more serious and require oral antibiotics—**never** ignore pain, redness, swelling, or discharge from a cartilage piercing, because they progress rapidly.
- Clean pierced jewelry weekly with alcohol or another antiseptic cleanser.
- Do **not** use alcohol or peroxide directly on your piercing site (although this used to be recommended, we now know that this actually irritates the skin and delays healing). Instead, clean the area by gently rubbing with a piece of gauze soaked with saline solution. Home recipe for saline solution: ½ teaspoon of salt in 1 cup of water.
- Dentists, orthodontists, and dental hygienists strongly recommend AGAINST any type of tongue piercings because of potential damage to teeth and gums. Tongue piercing risks include tooth chipping (most common problem), speech impairment, and drooling. Despite bacteria-laden mouths,

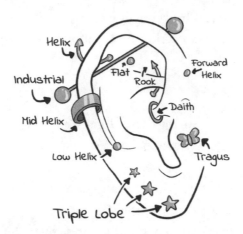

Helix

Flat

Rook

Forward Helix

Industrial

Daith

Mid Helix

Low Helix

Tragus

Triple Lobe

infections are surprisingly uncommon, though when they do occur, infections are potentially severe because they can block your airway.

o To minimize risks with nasal piercings, stick to the lateral nostril (rather than the central septum cartilage) and consider a seamless hoop to avoid the embedding issue of studs.

o Keloids are cosmetically disturbing, overly aggressive scar tissue that can occur with any piercing (or tattoo). Risk factors include having relatives with keloids, ages ten to thirty, and dark skin (fifteen times greater risk). See your doctor *as early as possible* if you begin to develop one of these raised scars after any piercing. Treatment is challenging, with many options, because there is not one "guaranteed" method, and early intervention improves outcomes.

Chapter 57
Thinking of Inking? Tattoos (Before and After)

What If: I Want Ink?
Medical Name: Tattoo

When did you decide?
Ideally, getting a tattoo is a well-thought-out decision made over the course of *at least* six months to a year, but we see a fair amount of Monday morning regret born of alcohol-fueled, impulsive birthday (*or Greek or graduation*) celebrations and/or peer-pressured choices.

What's the big deal? Can't you have tattoos easily removed?
No! Although ads for "laser tattoo removal" abound, removal does not equal "back to normal skin," and the process is predictably painful, expensive, and lengthy. Nothing "easy" about it.
- Tattoo removal typically requires a series of laser treatments every six to ten weeks over the course of a year or two (depending on size and colors), and average cost *per session* is two to five hundred dollars.

285

- Like tattooing, laser removal treatment also causes some bleeding, swelling, and pain, plus risk of infection and scarring.
- Small, black ink tattoos on light skin have the highest success rate, while brighter colors like yellow, white, or purple are extremely difficult to eliminate, especially on darker skin.
- Dermatologist Steve Mahoney, MD, notes, "Tattoos seem super cool . . . until they have to come off. My office is filled with people in their late thirties and early forties that want theirs removed, and many are pissed off at their teenage self—*especially when it's time to pay the bill.*"

What are the actual medical risks of tattoos?

Infection:
How common?

Honestly, we aren't sure because tattoo-related infections are not reportable. The medical literature focuses on severe infections and complications that occur less than 0.1 percent of the time, when contaminated ink, poor sterilizing techniques, or nonmedical wound care have led to hospitalization and/or death. Self-reported survey studies suggest a higher but still very low annual infection rate between 0.5 percent and 6.0 percent. My clinical experience in a highly inked town suggests minor tattoo-related skin infections are at least this common, but all agree that allergic and inflammatory reactions outweigh infections.

What type?

The most common type of tattoo-related infection is a bacterial (usually staph) infection that comes from either nonsterile technique at the tattoo parlor or, more commonly, *from scratching the fresh ink with your own unclean hands,* especially if you have a pronounced inflammatory reaction with multiple raw, bleeding areas within your new tattoo. If you contract the resistant strain of staph called MRSA (Methicillin Resistant Staph Aureus), this infection can be very challenging to treat.

With fresh ink, new needles, and sterile technique, the risk of contracting blood-borne viral infections like HIV and Hepatitis B are truly minimal. The same should be true for Hepatitis C, but for unknown reasons, studies still show Hep C being diagnosed up to four times more frequently in people with at least one tattoo, even taking into account other risk factors.

Inflammatory reactions:

The larger and more complex your new tattoo is, the higher the likelihood that you will experience temporary redness, pain, swelling, and oozing or bleeding for a couple weeks. You have a raw, open wound from a zillion needle pricks, so following strict aftercare is critical to avoid infection.

A minority of people will develop overly aggressive immune responses that lead to red bumps called granulomas (most commonly with red ink) or heaped-up scars called keloids, both significant cosmetic problems. Note that if you have any keloid scar on your body from previous trauma or surgery, your risk of the same with tattoos is significant.

Ink allergies:

Itch, rash, swelling, and irritation with sun exposure are common self-reported complaints about tattoos. **Red ink is the most common culprit** because of mercury sulfide, but all colors can produce an allergic reaction that creates itchy red bumps and swelling within or immediately next to the ink. Unfortunately, these allergic reactions can occur immediately or any time weeks or many years after getting a tattoo.

Yellow inks and some red inks contain cadmium sulfide, which can trigger an allergic reaction when exposed to sunlight. Look for itching, redness, swelling, blisters, and oozing or flaking skin concentrated around this color within your tattoo.

What else?

- If you already have or are genetically predisposed to skin disorders like psoriasis or eczema, getting a tattoo can trigger an initial outbreak or recurrent flares.

- Most people with one tattoo will get more ink (70 percent have more than one tattoo; 20 percent have more than five tats).

What about henna tattoos?

- Pure henna dye is a well-tolerated extract from a plant called *Lawsonia inermis,* and allergic reactions are extremely rare and mild.
- However, henna tattoos that look black (versus a reddish brown) have additives such as heavy metals and most commonly a hair dye called paraphenylenediamine (PPD), which can cause delayed but intense allergic reactions.
- This "black henna" (PPD) reaction is a contact dermatitis that emerges three to ten days after the tattoo is placed, usually appearing as itchy red bumps and blisters that ultimately scab and may cause permanent discoloration or scarring.
- With any contact dermatitis skin allergy (think poison ivy), you may not react the first time you are exposed to the agent, *but each subsequent exposure increases your chance of reaction if you are susceptible.* Likewise, being sensitized from a henna tattoo can make you allergic to hair color if that dye contains PPD. The good news is that only a small minority (roughly 6 percent) of North Americans react to the PPD dye in skin testing studies, and the chance of creating this contact allergy is estimated to be 2.5 percent per application of black henna tattoo ink.
- *Bottom line: Pure Henna tattoos without PPD are generally safe even with frequent reapplications, but black henna tattoos are discouraged.*

Treatment:

- **Most tattoo-related infections are mild** and can be treated with topical or oral antibiotics and strict wound care technique.
- **Allergic reactions** to tattoo ink are often managed with topical steroid creams or ointments, but more severe reactions may require oral steroids or, rarely, tattoo removal.

- **Sun exposure reactions** are typically managed with topical steroids and increasing physical barriers (clothing) over the tattoo.
- **Henna tattoo allergy treatment** includes oral antihistamines plus prescription topical and possibly oral steroids.

Head in to see your doctor if:
- Your tattoo or the surrounding area develops increasing swelling, rash, discharge, or pain.
- You develop whole-body symptoms like fever, nausea, chills, or body aches.
- You develop hives and/or shortness of breath.
- Sun exposure triggers transient red bumps, blisters, swelling, itch, or discomfort in one or more colors of your tattoo.

Deciding if your symptoms represent infection versus expected inflammation can be challenging—if you're unsure, get checked out!

Worst-case scenario:
Most common worst case is a poor cosmetic outcome due to scarring from wound infections, excessive scratching, allergic reactions, or abnormal healing (keloids and granulomas).

Only an estimated 0.02 percent of all tattoos end up causing severe infectious or allergic life-threatening complications.

Prevention of tattoo complications:
- Choose a licensed tattoo parlor (*if your state does that*) and look for excellent hygiene that includes autoclaving (sterilizing) all reusable equipment and wiping surfaces with bleach-containing cleansers between clients.
  - The tattoo artist should wash their hands thoroughly and wear latex gloves before touching you.
  - Fresh needles and ink should be opened from their packaging directly in front of you.

- In 2012, a multistate outbreak of tuberculous-like tattoo infections turned out to be from ink that was contaminated in the factory, so even fresh ink is not a 100 percent guarantee.
  - Tattoo ink is a cosmetic, not a drug, so the FDA has less regulatory control.
  - Communicate with your artist and your doctor if you develop any rash.
- *Aftercare is critical*, so discuss specifics with your artist but expect to:
  - Leave on initial bandage for five to twenty-four hours, then remove and leave ink uncovered.
  - Clean several times per day using an unscented mild antibacterial liquid soap, water, and your hands (no washcloths or scrubbers) and then rinse thoroughly and air-dry or pat dry with paper towels.
  - Apply a thin layer of nonscented petroleum-based ointment (like Aquaphor) to clean and dry tattoo after each cleaning.
  - Tattoo will start to scab and flake after several days to a week; *never pull off or pick at these* (cover loosely with clothing to remove temptation).
- As much as you want to show off your new tattoo, fresh ink must be covered if you are going to be out in the sun for at least the first three weeks.
- No pools, hot tubs, rivers, lakes, or oceans until fresh tattoo is fully healed (at least three weeks, probably longer).

TIPS:

- When you've decided on your tattoo, **start with a pure henna** (not black henna) version and then continue reapplications, tweaking the size/shape/content of your tattoo for at least six months, preferably a year. Yes, this is expensive and time-consuming, but not as costly, risky, or time-consuming as tattoo revision or removal.

○ Before you permanently ink, ask every "older" inked person (at least five years your senior) whom you encounter (store clerks, waiters, doctors, etc.) about their tats to **get first-hand feedback about the pros and cons** of the size, shape, location, color, and content of their ink. Fashions and personal tastes change faster than you think; odds are good something you adored in middle school or even high school now makes you cringe.

○ If your henna tattoo artist is painting with black ink or it only takes an hour to stain, this henna contains PPD and is risky. Natural henna paste is reddish orange and has to sit on your skin for at least several hours.

○ If you are getting ink writing in a different language, **confirm the spelling** with a native speaker; do not rely on your artist, *especially* with Chinese characters.

○ *Do not ink a name unless it's a family member or perhaps a loved one who passed away;* other names may not remain significant. "Names" are the number-one tattooing regret across socioeconomic boundaries.

○ Most job interviewers do not want to see your ink, so consider a body location that can easily be covered with business clothing.

Chapter 58
I Might Need Stitches (Cuts and Scrapes beyond Band-Aids)

What If: I Might Need Stitches? Cuts and Scrapes beyond Band-Aids?

Medical Name: Lacerations & Abrasions & Puncture Wounds

What most likely happened:

Scenario A: You and your fellow architect majors were working late into the night finishing a project when your hand slipped with the X-Acto knife, slicing into your finger or the top of your nondominant hand. Helpful friends grab paper towels to keep your blood off the project, and a grad student peeks at your finger and offers you superglue to seal your cut. (*I swear we hear this story once a week!*) Obviously, you can cut yourself a million other ways, but ultimately with any cut, you want to know if you need to be seen and/or stitched up. Take a minute to notice details: **What did you cut yourself with?** (The edge of a rusty metal fence? If you're in the kitchen, was the knife clean or had you been cutting up chicken?)

    Scenario B: Rushing to class on your bike in the rain, you swerve to avoid a texting pedestrian (or an oblivious scooter rider) and end up splayed across the gravel road—your palms, forearms, knees, and chin oozing with road rash and a deep gash near your knee from landing on your bike pedal.

Treatment:

- **Bleeding: Hold constant pressure** for at least five minutes, ideally using a clean towel or bandage; resist the temptation to peek frequently to "check" the bleeding.
- If possible, clean the wound by placing it under running water for several minutes and **wash, wash, wash**! *More flushing = cleaner wound, better healing.*
- Use liquid soap if handy, but **do not scrub**, and **do NOT use peroxide, iodine, or alcohol** (these cleansers actually damage the skin and delay healing).
- If stitches are needed, you've got a window of about six to eight hours (up to a max of twenty-four hours for some cuts) to decide; beyond that, the risk of infection outweighs the benefits of closure.

Head to your doctor immediately if:

- Holding pressure for ten minutes doesn't stop the bleeding.
- The bleeding is coming in spurts.
- Cut is near a joint (most commonly a knuckle or knee), through a (finger- or toe-) nail, or on your face or genitals.
- Obviously, if cut is large or deep or involves tendons or nerves (if you lose motion or sensation).
- There is "stuff" in the cut (rust, metal fragments, etc.).

For a cut that happened more than a day ago, head to the doctor if signs of infection:

- Increasing redness, swelling, tenderness
- Fever or chills
- Red streaks moving up from the cut

Does your cut need to be stitched, glued, or stapled?

If your cut is deeper than ¼ inch or longer than ¾ inch **or** if the cut gapes open so you have to push the sides together for them to touch, *you probably need your cut repaired by a clinician.*

- **Stitches:** Best suited for deep or jagged cuts, any cuts on mobile areas like fingers and other joints (because stitches hold stronger than the glue), plus the vast majority of cosmetically important areas (face, lips, around eyes, etc.)
- **Glue (Dermabond):** Best for simple, shallow, straight cuts on areas of skin that do not get pulled by motion from nearby joints
- **Staples:** Frequently used on scalp lacerations and other large cuts because they are faster and easier, but some studies show a greater risk of infection (versus stitches)

Can I use the OTC medical "superglue" from a drugstore?

The million-dollar question, right? Answer is **maybe** for simple, shallow, straight cuts that don't involve eyes, mouth, face, genitals, or joints . . . at your own risk. If you are going to use it, the time is when the cut happens, *not a day or two later.* Remember, the biggest problem is not cleansing the wound enough before sealing everything in below the glue, thus setting up a perfect spot for infection. Also know that glue is only for the skin layer; if you have cut into tendon, fat, or muscle, those must be repaired with suture.

Scraped hands and knees (a.k.a. road rash)
Three things to know:

1. Wash, wash, wash—use copious amounts of water and add liquid soap. **Avoid other cleansers** (like peroxide and alcohol). Take the time to find a bathroom and really cleanse rather than slapping a Band-Aid on over a dirty scrape and waiting till the end of the day to clean properly.
2. These are "dirty" wounds—a risk for tetanus. If it's been more than five years since your last tetanus booster (your record will say Td or Tdap), then you need a booster now.

3. Should you add some OTC triple antibiotic ointment? Nope! *Dermatologists no longer endorse antibiotic ointments as routine treatment to prevent infection for scrapes and cuts.* Instead, they recommend using a thin layer of petroleum jelly to keep the wound moist to promote healing. What's wrong with using OTC triple antibiotic ointment? Perhaps the largest deterrent is the fact that between 1 and 9 percent of the population will have an allergic reaction to the neomycin component, which shows up as an irritated, red contact dermatitis, often mistaken for a worsening infection. Additionally, antibiotic resistance is a growing problem, so we want to reduce all types of unnecessary use of antibiotics, and frankly, current evidence does not convincingly show that application of OTC antibiotic ointments isn't any more effective than simply using petroleum jelly. *Note that using a tube of petroleum jelly (rather than a tub) helps reduce the risk of spreading dirt or bacteria.*

Worst-case scenario:

You cut deep enough to damage an artery (that spurting bleeder), a tendon, or a nerve, and you will need surgery to fully correct the problem. More commonly, though, worst case is a cosmetic issue of an ugly scar. Perhaps you needed stitches but didn't want to go in, but decide a couple days later that the cut looks gross or infected, so you head to the doctor only to find out it's now too late for stitches (although we can certainly help with any infection).

Prevention:

- Slow down! Allow extra time to get to class on rainy/icy/cold days.
- Architect majors: Most accidents happen the final night of a project thanks to overcaffeinated, anxiety-filled rushing. Again, **slow down** or, better yet, resist the architecture procrastination stereotype (check out Tim Urban's "Ted Talk: Inside the Mind of a Procrastinator").

TIPS:

- o Using OTC craft superglue is risky and can actually cause chemical burns on your skin, especially if it comes into contact with cotton or other fabrics (like your pants), not to mention common complications like accidentally sticking your fingers together from drippy, runny superglue. Medical grade "superglue" is a different product that has antimicrobial properties and is less toxic to healthy skin.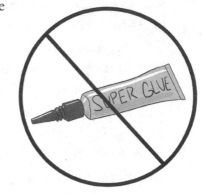

- o Using OTC medical "superglue" is more complicated than it sounds; read and follow all the instructions if you choose to self-treat a simple, shallow, straight cut. Never put creams or ointments (like antibiotic cream) on top of a wound closed with glue.

- o **Record the date of your last tetanus shot** (and which type, Tdap or Td) in your phone; boosters are needed every ten years, but we give boosters earlier for "dirty" wounds (cuts involving unclean surfaces) if it's been more than five years since your last booster.

- o **If you have redness** around your scrape or cut, **trace around the edge with a ballpoint pen**. If the redness goes outside of your marks the next day, you know infection is spreading and you should see your doctor.

- o Your best cosmetic result comes from the earliest intervention, so if you have any question about whether you need stitches, get seen within eight hours of your injury.

Chapter 59

Nail Issues: Infected, Ingrown, or Just Can't Stop Biting Them

What If: My Nail Looks Infected (and I Can't Stop Biting Them)?

Medical Name: Paronychia, Onychophagia, Ingrown Nail

What most likely happened:

Seems like your mom's been nagging you your whole life to stop biting your nails, but you never really cared until college. Your honors program orientation began with an advisor discussing key "real world" first impression tips—from appropriate business attire and a firm handshake down to hygiene details like clean, trimmed nails. Ironically, you were absentmindedly messing with a hangnail as he spoke, picking at a swollen, tender, red section of the side of your index finger.

What's going on?

Well, 44 percent of adolescents and 19 to 29 percent of young adults routinely bite their nails. This extremely common, persistent habit is largely a cosmetic issue or social frustration but may also cause a local skin infection or an abscess. All body-focused repetitive behaviors (BFRBs) like nail biting, hair pulling, and skin picking tend to run in families, though a specific genetic link is not yet identified. Additionally, there is association of nail biting with oral infections, dental enamel and root problems, and TMJ (temporomandibular joint syndrome). Nail biters typically mess with their nails when they are bored, nervous, or hungry. More rough edges or hangnails encourage more biting or tearing, further damaging the nails and perpetuating the problem.

Toenails are more often torn than bitten, though some flexible individuals continue to bite toenails into adulthood. Ingrown nails occur more in males, classically on the great toe. Ingrown nails typically start with an overly curved or torn nail that is too short along the lateral side, aggravated by constant pressure from tight footwear. This inflamed area allows surface bacteria and fungus inside, creating a skin infection or an abscess.

Treatment:

Nail biting is challenging to treat and best approached with multiple treatments:

- Bitter-tasting topical products (such as Mavala Stop) increase awareness for absent-minded biting.
- False nails or dip powder (SNS) are very effective (cannot be chewed through or torn) while in place (dip is preferred over gels because dip does not require UV lighting, which is a risk factor for skin cancer).
- Chewing gum may serve as an oral distraction.
- Wearing a rubber "bracelet" to "pick at" can be a soothing alternate behavior.
- Carry a fidget spinner, silly putty, or stress ball to squeeze.
- Mouth guards and retainers make it physically difficult to bite.
- Cognitive Behavioral Therapy (CBT)
    - Habit-Reversal Training (increases awareness of action and teaches an alternate response, such as immediately stretching out all your fingers for thirty seconds when you notice your hand on its way to your mouth)

- • Progressive Muscle Relaxation
- • Stimulus Control Therapy (focuses on identifying triggers)
- Medication: Fluoxetine (Prozac) or other SSRIs may help with nail biting.
- Medical assessment and blood tests: rule out causes for weakened, cracked, or splitting nails; thyroid deficiency or excess and B12 deficiency are common disorders that affect nail quality.

Infected fingernails can be extremely painful. Treatment starts with warm water soaks (twenty minutes, multiple times per day), and OTC antibiotic ointment may be applied. If pain, redness, or swelling increases, or if you see any pus, your doctor should examine your finger and will likely need to drain the abscess.

Early ingrown nail treatment includes:
- Frequent warm water soaks (four times a day for twenty minutes)
- Wear shoes with a wide toe box, no pressure on the toe.
- Slide a small piece of dental floss under the embedded corner to lift the nail edge; replace this floss daily.
- Topical antibiotic ointment may be applied to clean, dry nail.

More severely ingrown or infected nails require minor surgery to remove either the lateral portion of the nail or the entire nail. Repeat ingrown nails may also require removal of a portion of the nail bed to prevent the nail from growing back.

Head to your doctor if:
- The side of your nail becomes red, swollen, painful, or very tender to touch.
- Conservative home treatment for a few days hasn't helped.
- You need help stopping biting your nails.

Worst-case scenario:

Typically, these infections are minor with the worst case being a small abscess that must be drained or an ingrown nail that requires partial or full removal. Underlying diseases like diabetes can allow these infections to progress and become more serious.

Prevention:
- Use clippers to trim nails; cut toenails straight across (not curved).
- If you have very dry hands (like from frequent use of alcohol-based sanitizers), be sure to use moisturizing lotion.
- Get monthly manicures (home or salon).

TIPS:
- MANicures are for both women and men and do not require nail polish; many men prefer only "buffed" nails (no polish).
- Investing in weekly manicures for a few months helps maintain motivation to stop biting nails for many people.
- Use cuticle scissors to immediately remove hangnails (rather than pulling or biting them off).

Chapter 60

Spring Break Rashes: "No-See-Ums" of the Sea

What if: You Get a Swimmer's Rash?

Medical name: Cercarial Dermatitis

What most likely happened:

While swimming in a lake or the ocean (or perhaps as you are drying off after swimming), you may suddenly feel stings all over your arms, legs, or body. These stings are from the infamous "no-see-ums" of the sea or fresh water. Despite body surfing, wading, or snorkeling with others, you may be the only one who suddenly feels these invisible stings. Others may feel fine while swimming, but minutes, hours, or even a day later, they begin feeling that prickling sensation. In either case, once the stinging begins, you will likely see mosquito bite–looking itchy red bumps and swelling.

What's going on:

Swimmer's rashes have many common names, including ocean itch, sea lice, clam-digger's itch, duck itch, or sea bather's eruption, to name a few. These rashes develop when different types of larvae burrow into a human rather than their desired host.

- **Rash mostly under your swimsuit: "Ocean Itch" or "Sea Lice."** Oceans are home to jellyfish, sea anemones, and corals, all of which contain "stinging cells" (cnidocytes) that can be triggered by touch. Their tiny larvae float in large yet practically invisible swarms, most commonly near the warmer surface water. Unsuspecting waders can easily wander into one of these swarms, causing hundreds of larvae to get caught in and under their swimsuit fabric, which often leads, unfortunately, to hundreds of stings. While you may also have a few scattered stings on your arms or legs, the largest concentration of stings will be located under your swimsuit.

- **Rash mostly on your arms and legs: "Swimmer's Itch" or "Duck Itch."** Freshwater lakes and ponds contain parasitic Schistosome (flat worm) larvae from infected snails. As part of their life cycle, these larvae leave the snail in search of a waterfowl or mammal host. These larvae can accidentally burrow directly into swimmers' uncovered skin (leaving the swimsuit-covered skin largely unaffected.) However, these parasites cannot live, grow, or reproduce in human skin, so they quickly die. Interestingly, not everyone reacts to this larval invasion of their skin, but in an unlucky subset, the larvae trigger an allergic reaction that includes the stinging sensation, itch, swelling, and a variety of skin reactions (red bumps, pimple-looking pustules, blisters and/or discoloration). Although rare, people with more intense allergic reactions may also develop progressive symptoms of headache, body aches, stomach nausea, diarrhea, and fever.

Treatment:

If you start to feel stings while swimming, get out of the water immediately. If you feel stinging under your swimsuit, remove your suit as soon as physically (and socially) possible. Know that fresh water and/or friction may trigger the larvae to sting, so it's *extremely important to remove your swimsuit before jumping into a shower or spraying yourself.* Vinegar may neutralize the toxin and reduce additional stings—apply to your body, and then remember to rinse your swimsuit in the vinegar, as well.

Additional treatment is targeted at the allergic reaction:

- Cool compresses may help ease the itch or burn
- Consider taking an oral antihistamine such as diphenhydramine (Benadryl), fexofenadine (Allegra), loratadine (Claritin), or cetirizine (Zyrtec)
- Apply topical steroid cream or ointment on your torso or extremities (not on the face or genitals)

Is this rash contagious?

No. Each bump is an allergic reaction to a single larva burrowing into the skin, and the larva cannot be spread from one person's body to another. Please note, however, if you borrowed a wet swimsuit from a friend, any larva trapped in the suit material could certainly sting you. If you experience a swimmer's rash, clean your swimsuit with hot water and dry it thoroughly in a dryer . . . or toss it, and get a new suit.

How long does the rash last?

The rash typically lasts anywhere from several days to up to two weeks.

Head to your doctor if:

- You have any shortness of breath, trouble swallowing, lip swelling, chest pain or tightness, abdominal pain/nausea/vomiting, or dramatically increasing swelling or redness from your sea rash. The more often you experience this allergic rash, the more quickly your symptoms will develop. Remember, this is an *allergic* reaction, so in theory, a severe reaction could potentially be life-threatening (although extremely rare).
- You develop fever or other signs of infection (increasing local redness, swelling, or pain).
- Your dermatitis involves your face or genitals.
- Your rash is not improving with cool compresses and over-the-counter medications.

Worst-case scenario:

Happily, the typical worst case is that you have an itchy, ugly rash for a couple weeks, or that you develop a secondary skin infection (from scratching your rash) and require antibiotics for that infection.

Prevention:

Know the stinging seasons:

- Jellyfish larvae season runs from March to August (peaking April through July) in the Atlantic Ocean, Gulf of Mexico, and Caribbean Sea. Florida beaches often alert swimmers of stinging danger by posting purple warning flags when the swarms are especially heavy.
- In freshwater lakes and ponds, the Schistosome larvae season is thankfully limited primarily to the first four to six weeks in early summer, when the water is the warmest. Although you can catch swimmer's itch in literally every county in the United States, the most common sites are in Michigan, Wisconsin, and the Great Lakes region.

Tips:

o While swimming in the ocean, consider wearing a swimsuit that covers less of your body (bikini versus one piece) and skip the T-shirt, because the more fabric on your body, the greater area for the larvae to get trapped next to your skin and sting you. (Of course, once you are back on the beach, cover up so you don't get sunburned!)

o Avoid hanging out around the shoreline. If you are a strong swimmer enjoying a freshwater lake or pond, you are better off swimming in the deeper, cooler waters because the larvae prefer the warm, shallow water.

o Please don't feed the ducks or geese on the shoreline or docks, because they play a key part of the life cycle of the flat worms. More ducks and geese equal higher risk of swimmers' rash!

O Most importantly: *do not freak out if you develop swimmers' rash!* Consider this equivalent to getting a whole bunch of mosquito bites on a hike or camping trip—uncomfortably itchy, yes, but the bumps should go away within a week or two, and they won't cause long-term issues.

Chapter 61
"Bartender" or "Margarita" Dermatitis

What If: You Get an Unusual, Asymmetrical Rash on Sun-Exposed Skin?

Medical Name: Phytophotodermatitis and Post-inflammatory Hyperpigmentation

What most likely happened:

You accidentally spilled a margarita (or perhaps dripped lemon or lime juice as you squeezed a fruit slice) onto your skin while you were hanging out in the sun, triggering what is known as a *phytophotodermatitis* (*phyto* meaning "plant," *photo* meaning "sunlight," *dermatitis* meaning "skin inflammation"). Subsequently, you may develop an itchy, red, and possibly blistered streak or patch on your body that leaves a persistent dark discoloration after the initial irritation resolves.

What's going on:

Phytophotodermatitis occurs as an inflammatory response, triggered by light activating the plant substance psoralen, which may have been left on your skin from plants like limes, parsley, celery, and carrots. The intensity of the reaction depends upon three things: the amount of the substance spilled onto the skin, the concentration of psoralen in the plant, and the amount of UVA exposure. The burning, red, and occasionally blistering skin lesions only appear about one to three days after the light exposure, which is part of the reason people often cannot figure out what caused their rash (because they naturally assume it was something they did immediately before the rash appeared). For this reason, most people falsely attribute this skin reaction to having touched poison ivy or being bitten or stung by insects.

Post-inflammatory hyperpigmentation simply describes the darkening of the skin after it was inflamed. We see this with everything from surgical scars to over-scratched mosquito bites, and although it may occur in anyone, this hyperpigmented response is typically more common in patients with darker skin color.

Treatment:
- The primary initial treatment is cold compresses, topical steroid preparations, and oral pain relievers as necessary for the acute symptoms.
- Prescription topical steroids are primarily used during the first stage, where there may be bumps, blisters, and redness. "Post-inflammatory" hyperpigmentation is just that—after the inflammation—so steroids are of little use by the time this darkened skin is present.
- Prescription bleaching creams may be utilized to try and lighten the darkened skin, but the primary treatment is both time and prevention of additional sun exposure.

Is this rash contagious?
- No. This rash requires the combination of citrus juice on the skin and sun exposure, and therefore, it cannot be transmitted to other places on your body or to other people.

How long does this rash last?

Perhaps the most frustrating part of this rash is that the discoloration can last for weeks to many months. The acute phase, however, with red bumps or blisters, typically only lasts for several days.

Head to your doctor if:
- You have significant immediate pain, swelling, or blisters.
- You are concerned about persistent discoloration of your skin.

Worst-case scenario:

If you scratch your rash, you can end up with a secondary bacterial infection that requires topical or oral antibiotics. However, for most people, the worst-case is ending up with a cosmetically displeasing dark mark on your skin for many months.

Prevention:
- Sunscreen and shade! It takes a combination of UV radiation along with the plant substance psoralen to create this problem, so eliminating one or the other helps prevent any issues.
- Bartenders—especially those in poolside or other outdoor locations—may want to consider long sleeves and/or gloves to protect their skin as they slice citrus fruits for drinks.
- This rash is worsened by wet, sweaty skin and/or heat, so keep a towel handy to dry your skin and position yourself in the shade of an umbrella or other sun-blocking cover to help prevent this dermatitis.

Tips:
- Simply being aware that citrus juice on your skin can cause a problem is half the battle! Remember to immediately and carefully wash off any juice that spills or splatters onto your skin if you may be exposed to sunlight.

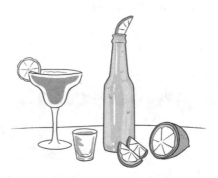

- The highest UVA levels occur in the middle of the day and at high altitude, so be extra careful in the midday sun and throughout the day on any mountain trips.
- Not surprisingly, the initial rash of red bumps and blisters may be misdiagnosed as a skin infection or a contact dermatitis like poison ivy, and kudos to your health-care provider if she or he can diagnose this problem when you come in only complaining of a dark streak or patch on your skin. Even though the rash typically starts with red bumps and blisters, many people only head to their doctor many weeks or months later, at which point they honestly may not recall how or when the discoloration began.

Bonus Section:
DIY First Aid Kit

First aid kits are wonderful graduation gifts! If you are crafty, have fun decorating your container using school colors, monograms, hand-drawn mascots, and enough ribbons to be Pinterest-worthy! If you're not, no worries—slap on a decal or use a red sharpie and put a red cross on it and call it done. It's the contents that really matter. Tackle box–style containers are my favorite, but "lunch boxes" and plain plastic shoe boxes work, too.

Suggested Contents:

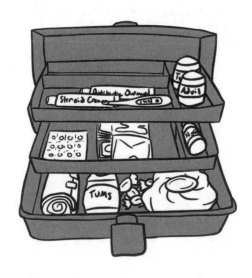

Include one item from each box. Name-brand examples are included for ease of recognition, but generics are perfectly fine, and trial-size or small quantities of each product keep the size of your kit reasonable. If you choose generic products, add an easily readable label with the most recognizable brand name.

Antihistamines:
- ☐ Nonsedating: Fexofenadine (Allegra) or Loratadine (Claritin) or Cetirizine (Zyrtec)
- ☐ Sedating: Diphenhydramine (Benadryl)
- ☐ Antivertigo, also sedating: Meclizine (Antivert, Bonine)

Nasal Steroid Spray:
- ☐ Fluticasone Propionate (Flonase) or Triamcinolone Acetonide (Nasacort)

Decongestant:
- ☐ Oxymetazoline nasal spray (Afrin)
- ☐ Oral pseudoephedrine (Sudafed)

Expectorant:
- ☐ Guaifenesin (Mucinex)

Cough Suppressant:
- ☐ Dextromethorphan (DM) liquid or capsules (Delsym or expectorant with DM, e.g., Mucinex DM)
- ☐ Cough drops of choice
- ☐ Combo product liquid or capsule "night-time cough reliever" (Nyquil or Robitussin)

Pain/Fever Relief: (*Yes, get all four—they have different uses*)
- ☐ Ibuprofen (Advil or Motrin)
- ☐ Naproxen (Aleve)
- ☐ Acetaminophen (Tylenol)
- ☐ Aspirin (Bayer)

Migraine Relief:
- ☐ Excedrin Migraine or Bayer Migraine: combinations of acetaminophen, aspirin, and caffeine

Topical Creams or Ointments:
- ☐ 1 percent Hydrocortisone Cream (Cortaid or Cortizone)
- ☐ Petroleum Jelly (Vaseline), Tube preferred over Tub
- ☐ Optional: Antibiotic Ointment
- ☐ Aloe and Lidocaine gels (Solarcaine, Alocaine, etc.)

Indigestion/heart burn:
- ☐ Antacid tablets: TUMS or Maalox (smooth dissolve)
- ☐ H2 Blockers: cimetidine (Tagamet HB), or famotidine (Pepcid AC or Zantac 360)
- ☐ PPI: omeprazole (Prilosec) or lansoprazole (Prevacid)

Diarrhea:
- ☐ Loperamide (Imodium)

Dehydration:
- ☐ Electrolyte replacement powder pack singles (Pedialyte, Liquid IV, etc.)

Eyes:
- ☐ Artificial tears: Blink, Systane, or Murine (not the "get the red out" ones)
- ☐ Small bottle of sterile saline eye wash

Miscellaneous:
- ☐ Naloxone nasal spray (Narcan OTC)
- ☐ Digital Thermometer (*choose like wine: not the cheapest, not the most expensive*)
- ☐ Spray Antiseptic Cleanser (such as Neosporin Wound Cleanser Foaming Liquid)
- ☐ Band-Aids: Be sure to include the "good ones": Blister, Knuckle and Fingertip bandages
- ☐ Throat lozenges/cough drops of choice
- ☐ Tweezers
- ☐ Cuticle scissors
- ☐ Ace Wraps (2—most students don't have these, so they disappear quickly!)

- ☐ Menthol topical analgesia cream or patch (such as Icy Hot, Bengay creams, or Salonpas patch)
- ☐ Reusable Ice Pack (the kind you fill with ice, because dorm freezer space is limited)
- ☐ Bulb Syringe (for ear irrigation)
- ☐ Roll of dog-poop bags (or other disposable trash bags) for convenient emesis (puke) bags and/or cleanup
- ☐ Heating pad (electric or microwaveable style)
- ☐ Condoms (*if you choose*)

TIPS:

- ○ **Antihistamine versus Decongestant:**
  - ○ **Itchy eyes, runny nose, sneezing?** Choose an antihistamine (nonsedating ones for daytime, sedating ones ok for evening).
    - ➢ *See: Chapter 24: Itching, Sneezing, Allergies, and Hives (page 128).*
  - ○ **Seasonal allergy symptoms** (above, plus congestion)? Use nasal steroid spray daily.
  - ○ **Stuffy nose or ear pressure?** Use any or all: nasal spray decongestant short term (<3 days), nasal steroid spray, and oral decongestant*

    *Oral phenylephrine is no longer recommended as of September 2023. Oral pseudoephredine is available without a prescription, but is regulated behind the counter, so you need to ask the pharmacist for this product
    - ➢ See Chapter 22: Stuffy Nose, Colds and Sinus Infections (page 117)
- ○ **Ibuprofen (Advil or Motrin) or Naproxen (Aleve) versus Acetaminophen (Tylenol)**
  - ○ **Ibuprofen & naproxen** are NSAIDs (Nonsteroid Anti-Inflammatory Drugs)
    - ➢ Both of these drugs decrease pain, lower fevers, and reduce swelling and inflammation.

- ➢ **Ibuprofen is the basic go-to pain reliever** (*unless you have stomach irritation, bleeding problems, or kidney issues, because NSAIDs make those worse*):
- ➢ Best choice for acute problems
    - ➢ Muscle aches, joint pain, strains, sprains, and swelling
    - ➢ High fevers
    - ➢ Oral/dental pain
- ➢ Ibuprofen is a "short-acting" NSAID, so it starts working sooner but wears off faster and will likely need repeat dosing.
- ➢ **Naproxen** is longer-acting—starts slower but lasts longer.
    - o Better choice for menstrual cramps and chronic conditions
- o **Acetaminophen (Tylenol):**
    - ➢ Reduces pain and lowers fevers.
    - ➢ Can potentially harm the liver but doesn't affect the kidneys, so avoid Tylenol if your liver might be inflamed (like from alcohol poisoning or infectious mono) and never exceed the recommended daily dose (six extra-strength caplets in twenty-four hours).
    - ➢ Works along different pathways than NSAIDs, so may be combined with ibuprofen if pain or fever not adequately improved with NSAIDs alone.
- o **Headache Pain Relief**
    - o If headache is on one side, throbbing, associated with light sensitivity and/or nausea:
        - ➢ OTC "Migraine" medication (these combine acetaminophen, aspirin, and caffeine)
        - ➢ OR take recommended dose of ibuprofen and/or acetaminophen and drink coffee or another caffeinated beverage.

➤ *See Chapter 2: Other Bad Headaches (Migraines) on page 8.*

○ If headache is on both sides, like a band around your head, constant pressure is

    ➤ Likely a tension or muscular headache, not migraine, so skip the caffeine and stick with ibuprofen and/or acetaminophen.

○ If it is from a hangover (or dehydration from a stomach virus with vomiting and diarrhea):

    ➤ Avoid acetaminophen (Tylenol).

    ➤ You may use ibuprofen (Advil) if not too nauseated.

    ➤ The real answer is rehydration: sip on electrolyte-fortified drinks (Pedialyte or a sports drink).

    ➤ *See Chapter 1: Hangovers on page 1.*

○ **Diarrhea Medications**

    ○ If you have a fever, do not try and stop the diarrhea (may prolong infectious diarrhea).

    ○ If you have occasional irritable bowel/test anxiety diarrhea: loperamide (Imodium)

    ○ After infectious diarrhea (from food poisoning or a stomach virus), stop all dairy products until your poop is back to normal for several days (because you are transiently lactose-intolerant).

    ○ Rehydrate with Pedialyte or sports drinks

        ➤ *See Chapter 37: Food Poisoning? Nausea, Vomiting, and Diarrhea on page 186.*

○ **Heartburn Medications**

    ○ Start with antacids for immediate relief (like TUMS smooth dissolve).

    ○ If symptoms persist for a few days, add an acid-blocking medication (H2 blockers like Pepcid or PPI like Prilosec), and if still not better, head to the doctor.

○ Most important, stop whatever you might be doing to increase stomach acid: alcohol, nicotine (including vaping), or taking too much ibuprofen (Advil).

> ➢ *See Chapter 40: College Is Giving Me Heartburn . . . or Maybe an Ulcer on page 202.*

○ **Hydrocortisone Cream (Cortizone, Cortaid, etc.)**

○ Steroids like hydrocortisone reduce itch and swelling—so use these topical creams and ointments for itchy, swollen skin problems like insect bites/stings or local allergic reactions (e.g., piercings).

○ Note that steroid creams can allow a skin infection (which may be red and itchy) to get worse, so if symptoms do not rapidly improve, head to the doctor.

○ *Intentionally not included: Although widely used, evidence is lacking to support use of topical antihistamines like diphenhydramine (Benadryl) creams, so I do not recommend them.*

○ **Petroleum Jelly versus Antibiotic Ointment**

○ Antibiotic ointments are no longer the "go-to" for cuts, scrapes, and "road rash"! We now restrict antibiotic ointment use for signs of infection (not as prevention) and generally prefer prescription antibiotic ointments that do not contain neomycin. Thoroughly wash your injury with copious water and a mild soap, then apply a thin layer of petroleum jelly and a Band-Aid. *Note that deep cuts, puncture wounds, bites, and burns need to be evaluated by a clinician, as you may also need other interventions like prescription antibiotics or a tetanus booster.*

> ➢ *See Chapter 58: I Might Need Stitches (Cuts and Scrapes beyond Band-Aids) page 292.*

○ **Thermometer Advice**

○ **Use it!** *Please, please, use it!* Knowing "how high" your temperature reached helps us diagnostically. *A true fever is a temperature greater than 100.5°F.*

- ○ Be sure you haven't had anything hot or cold to drink for about ten minutes before you check your temperature.
- ○ Check and record your temperature again when your medicine should be wearing off—roughly five to six hours for acetaminophen (Tylenol) and seven to eight hours for ibuprofen (Advil).
- ○ **Narcan OTC**
  - ○ As of September 2023, naloxone nasal spray no longer requires a prescription—be sure this is in your kit!
  - ○ Never hesitate to use this spray if you find someone unconscious because it will cause no harm and may save a life!
  - ○ Do not "prime the spray." There is only one dose in each unit.
  - ○ ALWAYS call 911 immediately after you administer Narcan.
    - ➤ See Chapter 10: One Pill Can Kill: How to Recognize and Treat Opioid (Fentanyl) Overdose (page 58)
- ○ **Check expiration dates** at the beginning of each semester!

About the Author

Jill Grimes, MD, grew up in a home where education and love of learning ruled supreme. Her dad, William Litzinger, PhD, a college professor and administrator, was so deeply devoted to his students (*and in fairness, to collegiate sports*) that the family requested guests wear university spirit attire to his memorial service. (*The family is convinced "Ye Old Prof" cheered from heaven, delighted with the vibrant sea of colorful jerseys.*) Dr. Grimes inherited her father's passion to work with young adults, making it a logical progression for her to move to college health when she was ready for a new challenge after more than two decades in private family practice. Truth be told, Dr. Grimes enjoys a special bond with her college student patients because they are the same age as her daughters, who are a thousand miles away in different directions for their own adventures. What's next? Dr. Grimes is excited be part of the team launching Thread Health, an innovative digital health platform for teens and young adults, with the ultimate goal of bringing more accessible health information and health care to at-risk teen youth.

Dr. Grimes is a proud Texas Aggie—a National Merit and Presidential Endowed Scholar from the class of 1987. She earned her medical degree at Baylor College of Medicine in 1991 and completed her Family Medicine residency training in Austin in 1994. Dr. Grimes cherished the relationships she maintained with her private practice patients, taking care of all ages, genders, and body parts. In 2008, her career expanded to include becoming a medical editor for the *5-Minute Clinical Consult*, and she also published her first book, *Seductive Delusions: How Everyday People Catch STDs* (Johns Hopkins University Press), which has been part of the high school curriculum in San Antonio, Texas, since 2010. Dr. Grimes loved giving back to the Harvard Medical School publishing course that launched her own second-chapter career by returning annually as a guest faculty member for roughly a decade. She enjoys teaching other doctors through the American Academy of Family Physicians and educating the lay public through speaking engagements, print media, online venues, and television and national radio talk shows. She is thrilled to bring the third edition of her passion project to life and wishes every student holding this book good health, wisdom, a strong work ethic, resilience when they stumble, and, ultimately, a diverse and successful collegiate experience!

Acknowledgments

verflowing thanks and gratitude go out first and foremost to my family—to Drew, the best husband on the planet, and our amazing daughters, Brittany and Nicole. I intended this book to be their high school graduation gift, so I'm a wee bit tardy . . . but it is dedicated with great love to our girls and their peers. Additionally, my mom heart is bursting with pride that Nicole is our illustrator (*not her first rodeo, but her first one with me!*). Thank you to the LMU animation department and to Tsehai Publishers for helping Nicole hone her skills. Thanks also to Disney and our favorite Mouse for continuing to shape Nicole's early career at Walt Disney World! We are equally proud of our daughter Brittany, who has earned her doctorate in Occupational Therapy at Washington University in St. Louis and has dedicated her career to helping students of all ages and abilities. I'm so lucky to be able to share some of her insights and tips with all of you!

To Julie Silver, MD, and the whole #HarvardWriters team, many thanks for all your continual support, critical feedback, and enthusiasm. Julie, this book hit my "sweet spot"!

Thank you to my amazing physician friends and colleagues who not only cheered me on, but also reviewed topics for medical accuracy and shared their "nuggets" of wisdom—especially Gretchen La Salle, MD; Kristyn Fagerberg, MD; Pranay Sinha, MD, Anne Liu, MD, Ayushi Chugh, MD Stephen Mahoney, MD; Julia Sargent, MD; Lauren Streicher, MD; Sanjiv Chopra, MD; and my forever hero, Frank Domino, MD.

To my village, friends, and chosen family (many of whom overlap with my doctor tribe), thank you for holding me accountable, cheerleading, and supporting me in every way. Special shout-outs to Lynn Lampert; Coni Butler; Lorna Belk; Gretchen La Salle, MD; Kristyn Fagerberg, MD; Julia Sargent, MD; Daniela Knight, MS, RD, LD; and Dana Corriel, MD. To my dear friend Shelly Dawson, fellow mom of past and present college students and BFF extraordinaire, an enormous thank-you for reading every single word of this book and offering fabulous editorial feedback.

Thank you to my wonderful agent, Jeanne Fredericks, who immediately understood why a book like this is needed, and to editor Nicole Frail, for enthusiastically jumping on board and working so hard on this project. As I pass this manuscript forward, I know our book is in excellent hands.

References

A Systematic Review on the Efficacy of Topical Acyclovir . . . https://emj
.europeanmedical-group.com/wp-content/uploads/sites/2/2018/10/A
-Systematic-Review-on-the-Efficacy-of-Topical-Acyclovir-Penciclovir
-and-Docosanol-for-the-Treatment-of-Herpes . . . .pdf.

"ACOG and SMFM Recommend COVID-19 vaccination for Pregnant
Individuals." *ACOG*. (n.d.). Retrieved September 9, 2021, from https://
www.acog.org/news/news-releases/2021/07/acog-smfm-recommend-
covid-19-vaccination-for-pregnant-individuals.

Advanced Solutions International, Inc. "Home: American College Health
Association (ACHA)." *ACHA*, https://www.acha.org/.

Advanced Solutions International, Inc. "National College Health
Assessment (NCHA)." *NCHA Home*, https://www.acha.org/NCHA.

American College Health Association, "National College Health Assessment
ACHA-NCHA III (Fall 2019-Spring 2023)," https://www.acha.org
/NCHA/ACHA-NCHA_Data/Publications_and_Reports/NCHA
/Data/Reports_ACHA-NCHAIII.aspx

Arria AM, Caldeira KM, Bugbee BA, Vincent KB, O'Grady KE. "The
academic consequences of marijuana use during college." *Psychol Addict
Behav*. 2015 Sep;29(3):564-75. doi: 10.1037/adb0000108. Epub 2015
Aug 3. PMID: 26237288; PMCID: PMC4586361.

Al-Momani H, Aolymat I, Almasri M, Mahmoud SA, Mashal S. "Prevalence
of gastro-intestinal symptoms among COVID-19 patients and the
association with disease clinical outcomes." *Future Sci OA*. 2023 Apr

21;9(5):FSO858. doi: 10.2144/fsoa-2023-0040. PMID: 37180610; PMCID: PMC10167716.

Barton, Christian, et al. "Patellar Taping for Patellofemoral Pain: A Systematic Review and Meta-Analysis to Evaluate Clinical Outcomes and Biomechanical Mechanisms." *British Journal of Sports Medicine*, vol. 48, no. 6, May 2013, pp. 417–424, doi:10.1136/bjsports-2013-092437.

Brown J, Farquhar C, Lee O, Toomath R, Jepson RG. "Spironolactone versus placebo or in combination with steroids for hirsutism and/or acne." Cochrane Database Syst Rev. 2009 Apr 15;(2):CD000194. doi: 10.1002/14651858.CD000194.pub2. PMID: 19370553.

Bryant, Richard R., et al. "The Effect of Drug Use on Wages: A Human Capital Interpretation." *The American Journal of Drug and Alcohol Abuse*, vol. 26, no. 4, 2000, pp. 659–682, doi:10.1081/ada-100101901.

Cantor, David, et al. "Report on the AAU Campus Climate Survey on Sexual Assault and Sexual Misconduct."(2015): 13.

Cascio Rizzo, A., Paolucci, M., Altavilla, R., Brunelli, N., Assenza, F., Altamura, C., & Vernieri, F. (2017). "Daith piercing in a case of Chronic Migraine: A Possible Vagal modulation." Frontiers in *Neurology, 8.* https://doi.org/10.3389/fneur.2017.0062

"CDC Reports on Latest Estimates of HSV-1, HSV-2 Prevalence in the United States." *Infectious Disease Advisor*, 18 Feb. 2019, https://www.infectiousdiseaseadvisor.com/home/topics/sexually-transmitted-diseases/cdc-reports-on-latest-estimates-of-hsv-1-hsv-2-prevalence-in-the-united-states/.

Center for Drug Evaluation and Research. "Information about the Risk of Blood Clots in Women Taking Drospirenone." *U.S. Food and Drug Administration*, FDA, https://www.fda.gov/drugs/drug-safety-and-availability/fda-drug-safety-communication-updated-information-about-risk-blood-clots-women-taking-birth-control.

Chong LY, Head K, Hopkins C, Philpott C, Burton MJ, Schilder AG. "Different types of intranasal steroids for chronic rhinosinusitis." Cochrane Database Syst Rev. 2016 Apr 26;4(4):CD011993. doi: 10.1002/14651858.CD011993.pub2. PMID: 27115215; PMCID: PMC8939045.

Commissioner, O. of the. (n.d.). *FDA requests removal of All Ranitidine PRODUCTS (ZANTAC) from the market.* U.S. Food and Drug Administration. Retrieved September 9, 2021, from https://www.fda.gov/news-events/press-announcements/fda-requests-removal-all-ranitidine-products-zantac-market.

Cropsey, Karen L., et al. "Mixed-Amphetamine Salts Expectancies among College Students: Is Stimulant-Induced Cognitive Enhancement a Placebo Effect?" *Drug and Alcohol Dependence*, vol. 178, 2017, pp. 302–309, doi:10.1016/j.drugalcdep.2017.05.024.

Delost, Gregory R., et al. "The Impact of Chocolate Consumption on Acne Vulgaris in College Students: A Randomized Crossover Study." *Journal of the American Academy of Dermatology*, vol. 75, no. 1, 2016, pp. 220–222, doi:10.1016/j.jaad.2016.02.1159.

Dieckmann, Ralf, et al. "The Risk of Bacterial Infection After Tattooing." *Deutsches Aerzteblatt Online*, July 2016, doi:10.3238/arztebl.2016.0665.

Fares, Jawad, et al. "Musculoskeletal Neck Pain in Children and Adolescents: Risk Factors and Complications." *Surgical Neurology International*, vol. 8, no. 1, 2017, p. 72, doi:10.4103/sni.sni_445_16.

Fontenelle, Leonardo Ferreira, and Thiago Dias Sarti. "Kidney Stones: Treatment and Prevention." *American Family Physician*, U.S. National Library of Medicine, 15 Apr. 2019, https://www.ncbi.nlm.nih.gov/pubmed/30990297?dopt=Abstract.

Gaitonde, David Y., et al. "Patellofemoral Pain Syndrome." *American Family Physician*, 15 Jan. 2019, https://www.aafp.org/afp/2019/0115/p88.html.

Grimes, Jill. *Seductive Delusions: How Everyday People Catch STIs*. Johns Hopkins University Press, 2016.

Horak, P., Mikeš, L., Lichtenbergová, L., Skála, V., Soldánová, M., & Brandt, S.V. (2015). "Avian Schistosomes and Outbreaks of Cercarial Dermatitis." *Clinical Microbiology Reviews*, 165-190. Retrieved from https://journals.asm.org/doi/pdf/10.1128/cmr.00043-14

Huisman S, van der Bent SAS, Maijer KI, Tio DCKS, Rustemeyer T. "Cutaneous non-allergic complications in tattoos: An overview of the literature." *Presse Med.* 2020 Dec;49(4):104049. doi: 10.1016/j. lpm.2020.104049. Epub 2020 Aug 5. PMID: 32768612.

Infographic-Marijuana Use and Prescription Drug . . . - Dea.gov. https: //www.dea.gov/sites/default/files/2018-07/Infographic_ MarijuanaUse_Prescription Drug MisUse_College (1).pdf.

Islam PS, Chang C, Selmi C, Generali E, Huntley A, Teuber SS, Gershwin ME. "Medical Complications of Tattoos: A Comprehensive Review." *Clin Rev Allergy Immunol.* 2016 Apr;50(2):273-86. doi: 10.1007/ s12016-016-8532-0. PMID: 26940693.

Jamet, E., Gonthier, C., Cojean, S., Colliot, T., & Erhel, S. (2020, January 18). "Does multitasking in the classroom affect learning outcomes? A naturalistic study." *Computers in Human Behavior.* Retrieved September 9, 2021, from https://www.sciencedirect.com/science/article/abs/pii/ S0747563220300200?via%3Dihub.

"Joint statement regarding Covid-19 vaccine in men desiring fertility from the society for male reproduction and urology (SMRU) and the society for the study of male reproduction" (SSMR). ASRM. (n.d.). Retrieved September 9, 2021, from https://www.asrm.org/news-and-publications /covid-19/statements/joint-statement-regarding-covid-19-vaccine-in -men-desiring-fertility-from-the-society-for-male-reproduction-and -urology-smru-and-the-society-for-the-study-of-male-reproduction -ssmr/.

Jayakody, Kaushadh, et al. "Exercise for Anxiety Disorders: Systematic Review." *British Journal of Sports Medicine*, Centre for Reviews and Dissemination (UK), Feb. 2014, https://www.ncbi.nlm.nih.gov/pubmed /23299048.

"Journal of Voice." *Journal of Voice | Vol 31, Issue 1, Pages A1-A16, 1-132 (January 2017) | ScienceDirect.com*, https://www.sciencedirect.com /journal/journal-of-voice/vol/31/issue/1.

Kaestner, Robert. "The Effect of Illicit Drug Use on the Wages of Young Adults." *Journal of Labor Economics*, vol. 9, no. 4, 1991, pp. 381–412, doi:10.1086/298274.

Klein, Peter A., and Richard A. F. Clark. "An Evidence-Based Review of the Efficacy of Antihistamines in Relieving Pruritus in Atopic

Dermatitis." *Archives of Dermatology*, vol. 135, no. 12, Jan. 1999, doi: 10.1001/archderm.135.12.1522.

Kucharska, Alicja, et al. "Significance of Diet in Treated and Untreated Acne Vulgaris." *Advances in Dermatology and Allergology*, vol. 2, 2016, pp. 81–86, doi:10.5114/ada.2016.59146.

Lakhan, Shaheen E., and Annette Kirchgessner. "Prescription Stimulants in Individuals with and without Attention Deficit Hyperactivity Disorder: Misuse, Cognitive Impact, and Adverse Effects." *Brain and Behavior*, vol. 2, no. 5, 2012, pp. 661–677, doi:10.1002/brb3.78.

Lalanne, Laurence, et al. "Acute Impact of Caffeinated Alcoholic Beverages on Cognition: A Systematic Review." *Progress in Neuro-Psychopharmacology and Biological Psychiatry*, vol. 76, 2017, pp. 188–194, doi:10.1016/j.pnpbp.2017.03.007.

Lawn W, Trinci K, Mokrysz C, Borissova A, Ofori S, Petrilli K, Bloomfield M, Haniff ZR, Hall D, Fernandez-Vinson N, Wang S, Englund A, Chesney E, Wall MB, Freeman TP, Curran HV. "The acute effects of cannabis with and without cannabidiol in adults and adolescents: A randomised, double-blind, placebo-controlled, crossover experiment." *Addiction*. 2023 Jul;118(7):1282-1294. doi: 10.1111/add.16154. Epub 2023 Feb 26. PMID: 36750134; PMCID: PMC10481756.

Logue JK, Franko NM, McCulloch DJ, et al. "Sequelae in adults at 6 months after COVID-19 infection." *JAMA Netw Open*. 2021;4:e210830. Erratum in: *JAMA Netw Open*. 2021;4:e214572. Accessed July 8, 2021. Article full text. https://jamanetwork.com/journals/jamanetworkopen/fullarticle/2776560

Ma, David. "Temporary Henna Tattoos May Lead to Permanent Problems." *AAP Gateway*, American Academy of Pediatrics, 1 Dec. 2009, https://www.aappublications.org/content/30/12/28.4.

MacDougall, C. & Maston, M. (2023) "Student perceptions of cannabis use," *Journal of American College Health*, 71:4, 1003-1017, DOI: 10.1080/07448481.2021.1910272

Marinho, Anna Carolina Ferreira, et al. "Fear of Public Speaking: Perception of College Students and Correlates." *Journal of Voice*, vol. 31, no. 1, 2017, doi:10.1016/j.jvoice.2015.12.012.

"Masks & face coverings for the public." IDSA Home. (2021, July 28). Retrieved September 9, 2021, from https://www.idsociety.org/covid -19-real-time-learning-network/infection-prevention/masks-and-face -coverings-for-the-public/?fbclid=IwAR19TJsxnmIGBfHm2vA0VQK 1_5eDkftWpAcjV4dFMqrjmiCQUsdoxRHWRg0

"Monitoring the Future: 2022 National Survey Results on Drug Use 1975– 2022." The University of Michigan Institute for Social Research, https: //monitoringthefuture.org/wp-content/uploads/2022/12/mtf2022.pdf

Morris, Marcia. *The Campus Cure: a Parents Guide to Mental Health and Wellness for College Students*. Rowman & Littlefield, 2018.

McQuillan G, Kruszon-Moran D, Flagg EW, Paulose-Ram R. "Prevalence of Herpes Simplex Virus Type 1 and Type 2 in Persons Aged 14-49: United States, 2015-2016." NCHS Data Brief. 2018 Feb;(304):1-8. PMID: 29442994.

National Institute on Drug Abuse. "Introduction." *NIDA*, https://www .drugabuse.gov/publications/research-reports/tobacco-nicotine-e -cigarettes/introduction.

National Institute on Drug Abuse, https://nida.nih.gov/news-events /news-releases/2023/08/marijuana-and-hallucinogen-use-binge-drinking -reached-historic-highs-among-adults-35-to-50

Niloy N, Hediyal TA, Vichitra C, Sonali S, Chidambaram SB, Gorantla VR, Mahalakshmi AM. "Effect of Cannabis on Memory Consolidation, Learning and Retrieval and Its Current Legal Status in India: A Review." *Biomolecules*. 2023 Jan 12;13(1):162. doi: 10.3390/biom13010162. PMID: 36671547; PMCID: PMC9855787.

Parasher, Gulshan, and Gregory L. Eastwood. "Smoking and Peptic Ulcer in the Helicobacter Pylori Era." *European Journal of Gastroenterology & Hepatology*, vol. 12, no. 8, 2000, pp. 843–853, doi:10.1097/00042737-200012080-00003.

Patel, Deepak S., et al. "Stress Fractures: Diagnosis, Treatment, and Prevention." *American Family Physician*, 1 Jan. 2011, https://www.aafp .org/afp/2011/0101/p39.html.

Patellar Taping for Patellofemoral Pain: a Systematic . . . http://www.rcsi.ie/files /facultyofsportsexercise/20141013101131_Patellar taping for patellofem .pdf.

Paulus DJ, Zvolensky MJ. "The prevalence and impact of elevated anxiety sensitivity among hazardous drinking college students." *Drug Alcohol Depend.* 2020 Apr 1;209:107922. doi: 10.1016/j.drugalcdep.2020.107922. Epub 2020 Feb 15. PMID: 32088590; PMCID: PMC7536785.

Peng, Fen, et al. "Henna Tattoo." *Chinese Medical Journal*, vol. 130, no. 22, 2017, pp. 2769–2770, doi:10.4103/0366-6999.218003.

Prevalence of Herpes Simplex Virus Type 1 and Type 2 in . . . https://www.cdc .gov/nchs/data/databriefs/db304.pdf.

Radin JM, Quer G, Ramos E, et al. "Assessment of prolonged physiological and behavioral changes associated with COVID-19 infection." *JAMA*, 2021;4:e2115959. Accessed July 8, 2021. Article full text. https://jama network.com/journals/jamanetworkopen/fullarticle/2781687

Rossheim, Matthew E., et al. "Electronic Cigarette Explosion and Burn Injuries, US Emergency Departments 2015–2017." *Tobacco Control*, vol. 28, no. 4, 2018, pp. 472–474, doi:10.1136/tobaccocontrol -2018-054518.

Simplot, Timothy C., and Henry T. Hoffman. "Comparison between Cartilage and Soft Tissue Ear Piercing Complications." *American Journal of Otolaryngology*, vol. 19, no. 5, 1998, pp. 305–310, doi:10.1016 /s0196-0709(98)90003-5.

Sosin, Michael, et al. "Transcartilaginous Ear Piercing and Infectious Complications: A Systematic Review and Critical Analysis of Outcomes." *The Laryngoscope*, vol. 125, no. 8, 2015, pp. 1827–1834, doi:10.1002/lary.25238.

"Stubborn Acne? Hormonal Therapy May Help." *American Academy of Dermatology*, https://www.aad.org/public/diseases/acne-and-rosacea /stubborn-acne/hormonal-therapy-may-help-stubborn-acne.

"Supplemental Material for The Academic Consequences of Marijuana Use During College." *Psychology of Addictive Behaviors*, 2015, doi:10.1037 /adb0000108.supp.

Swift R, Davidson D. "Alcohol hangover: mechanisms and mediators." *Alcohol HEALTH Res World.* 1998;22(1):54-60. PMID: 15706734; PMCID: PMC6761819.

Titus, Stephen, and Joshua Hodge. "Diagnosis and Treatment of Acne." *American Family Physician*, 15 Oct. 2012, https://www.aafp.org /afp/2012/1015/p734.html#afp20121015p734-b20.

van Lawick van Pabst AE, Devenney LE, Verster JC. "Sex Differences in the Presence and Severity of Alcohol Hangover Symptoms." *J Clin Med.* 2019 Jun 17;8(6):867. doi: 10.3390/jcm8060867. Erratum in: J Clin Med. 2019 Aug 26;8(9): PMID: 31213020; PMCID: PMC6617014.

Verster JC, Slot KA, Arnoldy L, van Lawick van Pabst AE, van de Loo AJAE, Benson S, Scholey A. "The Association between Alcohol Hangover Frequency and Severity: Evidence for Reverse Tolerance?" *J Clin Med.* 2019 Sep 21;8(10):1520. doi: 10.3390/jcm8101520. PMID: 31546619; PMCID: PMC6832275.

U.S. Department of Health and Human Services. "Smoking Cessation. A Report of the Surgeon General." Atlanta, GA: U.S. Department of Health and Human Services, Centers for Disease Control and Prevention, National Center for Chronic Disease Prevention and Health Promotion, Office on Smoking and Health, 2020.

Wallach, Helene S., et al. "Virtual Reality Cognitive Behavior Therapy for Public Speaking Anxiety." *Behavior Modification*, vol. 33, no. 3, Nov. 2009, pp. 314–338, doi:10.1177/0145445509331926.

Wang B, Liu ST, Rostron B, Hayslett C. "Burn injuries related to E-cigarettes reported to poison control centers in the United States, 2010-2019." *Inj Epidemiol.* 2020 Jul 20;7(1):36. doi: 10.1186/s40621-020-00263-0. PMID: 32684171; PMCID: PMC7370415.

Warren, Terri. *The Good News about the Bad News: Herpes, Everything You Need to Know.* New Harbinger, 2009.

Xie, Yanfei, et al. "Prevalence and Risk Factors Associated with Musculoskeletal Complaints among Users of Mobile Handheld Devices: A Systematic Review." *Applied Ergonomics*, vol. 59, 2017, pp. 132–142, doi:10.1016/j.apergo.2016.08.020.

Zambrano LD, Ellington S, Strid P, et al. "Update: Characteristics of Symptomatic Women of Reproductive Age with Laboratory-Confirmed SARS-CoV-2 Infection by Pregnancy Status –United States, January 22-October 3, 2020." *MMWR Morb Mortal Wkly Rep* 2020; 69:1641-1647. DOI: http://dx.doi.org/10.15585/mmwr.mm6944e3

Index